LYME DISEASE

Edited by **Ali Karami**

Lyme Disease
Edited by Ali Karami

Published by InTech
Janeza Trdine 9, 51000 Rijeka, Croatia

Publishing Process Manager Vedran Greblo

Technical Editor Teodora Smiljanic

Cover Designer InTech Design Team

Additional hard copies can be obtained from orders@intechopen.com

Lyme Disease, Edited by Ali Karami
p. cm.
ISBN 978-953-51-0057-7

For EU product safety concerns:
IN TECH d.o.o., Prolaz Marije Krucifikse Kozulić 3, 51000 Rijeka, Croatia,
info@intechopen.com or visit our website at intechopen.com.

Meet the editor

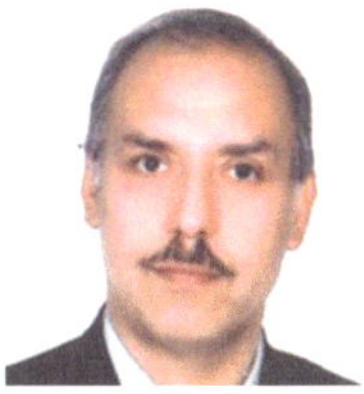

Dr Ali Karami was born in Tehran, Iran in 1957. He is Associate Professor of Molecular Biology and Genetic Engineering and is a Medical Biotechnology expert at the Research Center of Molecular Biology, Baqiyatallah University of Medical Sciences. He received his PhD in 1996 from Copenhagen University Faculty of Medical Science in Denmark. Since 1991 he has been working on the molecular biology of Borrelia burgdorferi with gene cloning and protein expression for Lyme disease recombinant vaccine and other infectious disease agents. He has published several books and numerous articles in national and international journals. He is currently head of Microarray Research Group and working on rapid molecular detection technologies, recombinant proteins, DNA vaccines and bioinformatics.

Contents

Preface

I began to work with Borrelia burgdorferi (Bb), the causative agent of Lyme disease or Lyme borreliosis, during my PhD at the University of Copenhagen in Denmark. In 1991 I was looking for an interesting research proposal to learn more about the molecular genetics world of infectious disease agents.

My advisor shared information about the complex structure of Borrelia spirochetes and the diseases they cause. Therefore, I started my experimental work in the Panum Institute with the culturing of Bb in a very specific culture medium. I extracted the smallest one mega base genome that is mostly linear compared to the circular genomes of most other microorganism. Two interesting phenomenon were observed about Bb. The one was that it contained more than a dozen extrachromosomal DNA elements or plasmids that were mostly linear. The other interesting finding was that this linear genetic structure had telomeres at the ends, like eukaryotic genomes.

I studied the genetic structure and molecular aspects of Bb mostly on molecular detection. I went on to study diagnosis and protection against the diseases by recombinant vaccines and subsequently published my papers on the subject, while contemplating writing a book on this agent.

Lyme disease is an emerging infectious disease characterized by skin changes, joint inflammation, and flu-like symptoms caused by the bacterium Borrelia burgdorferi transmitted by the bite of a deer tick. Early symptoms may include fever, headache, fatigue, depression, and a characteristic circular skin rash called erythema migrans. Symptoms resolve in three to four weeks even without treatment, but secondary or tertiary disease may develop if the initial infection is not treated. The symptoms may affect the joints, heart, and central nervous system. In most cases, the infection and its symptoms are eliminated by antibiotics, especially if the illness is treated early. Delayed or inadequate treatment can lead to the more serious symptoms, which can be disabling and difficult to treat.

Although Allen Steere realized in 1978 that Lyme disease was a tick-borne disease, the cause of the disease remained a mystery until 1981 when B. burgdorferi was identified by Willy Burgdorfer.

Lyme disease diagnosis and treatment is hampered by the lack of biological markers and no standardized treatment protocols. The treatment of patients is hampered by the fact that no combination of antibiotics completely eradicates the infection, which can then posture as a self-perpetuating autoimmune response in the patient. There are over 100 strains of Borrelia burgdorferi in the US, and 300 strains worldwide.

An interesting opportunity was presented to me in 2011 by Intech – Open Access Publisher to write a book about Lyme disease. With the collaboration of scientists around the world we started to prepare the chapters. It took over a year to finalize the book.

This book presents an overview of new diagnosis and treatment protocols arising from current research. The addressed topics include the pathophysiology of Lyme disease, antigenic variability, co-infection of other tick-borne diseases, the mechanisms that allow the spirochete to evade the immune system, the lack of response to antibiotic treatment, differential diagnosis of rheumatological, and neurological conditions.

In chapter one, the molecular biology of the Lyme disease agent is discussed in detail with regards to genome organization with interesting linear and circular plasmids. In chapter two, zoonotic peculiarities of Borrelia burgdorferi is discussed. Chapters three and four cover detection, diagnosis, advancement in Borrelia burgdorferi antibody testing, and the serology diagnostic schemes in Bb. Chapter five discusses the discovery of Lyme disease in ticks and dogs. In chapter six you will read about adaptation to glucosamine starvation in Bb. The final chapter covers porins in the genus Borrelia.

This book will be of use to medical doctors, clinicians, biologists and physicians specializing in the treatment of Lyme disease.

I would like to extend my sincere appreciation and thanks to Professor Benz Roland, Professor Nelson David, Dr Movila Alexandru, Dr Lakos András, Dr Tokarska-Rodak Małgorzata, Dr Savic Sara, also special thanks to Igor Babic as publishing process manager and my special gratitude to Intech – Open Access Publisher for their encouraging support in the publication of this book.

Ali Karami
Research Center of Molecular Biology
Baqyiatallh University of Medical Sciences, Tehran,
Iran

1

Molecular Biology of *Borrelia burgdorferi*

Ali Karami
Research Center of Molecular Biology, Baqyiatallah University of Medical Sciences, Tehran Iran

1. Introduction

Borrelia may be unique among prokaryote in having a genome that is mainly linear DNA physical and genetic map of linear chromosome of *B. burgdurferi* has been published, it consist of 946 to 952 kb Linear DNA (Sherwood *et al*;1993, Davidson *et al*;1992, Barbour *et al*; 1982).

This bacteria also contains several circular and specially linear plasmids from 5 to 55 kb. Recently analysis of entire *Agrobacterium tumefaciens* C58 genome revealed presence of one 2.1-Mb linear and one 3- Mb circular plasmid (Servent *et al*; 1993) and it has been shown that *rhodococcus fascians* contains 4 Mb linear chromosome (Crespi *et al*; 1992). Presence of several linear plasmids seems the segmentation of *Borrelias* DNA to several linear pieces has led to the suggestion that the relatively small linear chromosome and the linear plasmids actually are minichromosoms. In *B. hermsii* it has been shown that total cellular DNA organized into several complete gnomes (*Kitten et al*; 1992) and it suggests that linear plasmids are like small chromosomes (Ferdows *et al*; 1989). Plasmid profile of B. *burgdorferi* from different geographical area has been revealed significant heterogeneity a feature that can be used for classification of bacteria within given species (Barbour *et al*; 1987, 1989). Another related spirochete *B. hermsii* like *B. burgdorferi* has several linear and circular plasmids and the genes responsible for antigenic variation are located in linear plasmids. In *B. burgdorferi* a 49 kb linear plasmid carries the genes for Outer Surface Protein A and B (OspA and OspB) (Barbour *et al*; 1987, Baril *et al*; 1989). It has been shown that passage of *B. burgdorferi* in BSK medium changes the plasmid profile and loss of plasmids may change the infectivity of organism (Schwan *et al; 1988*, Simpson, *et al*; 1990). Structure of Linear plasmids of *B. burgdorferi* shows similarity to eukaryotic virus such as vaccinia and African swine fever virus in having covalently closed ends like hairpin loops (Hinnebusch *et al*; 1991).

1.1 Taxonomy and classification

Borrelia burgdorferi belongs to the phylum Spirochaetes. The members of this phylum are long, thin, helically coiled bacteria that have flagella (*axial filaments*) running lengthwise between the peptidoglycan layer and the outer membrane. Movement of the flagellum produces a screw-like motion that propels the organism.

The phylum Spirochates contains a single class (Spirochaetes), a single order (Spirochaetales), and three families: Brachyspiraceae, Leptospiraceae, and Spirochaetaceae.

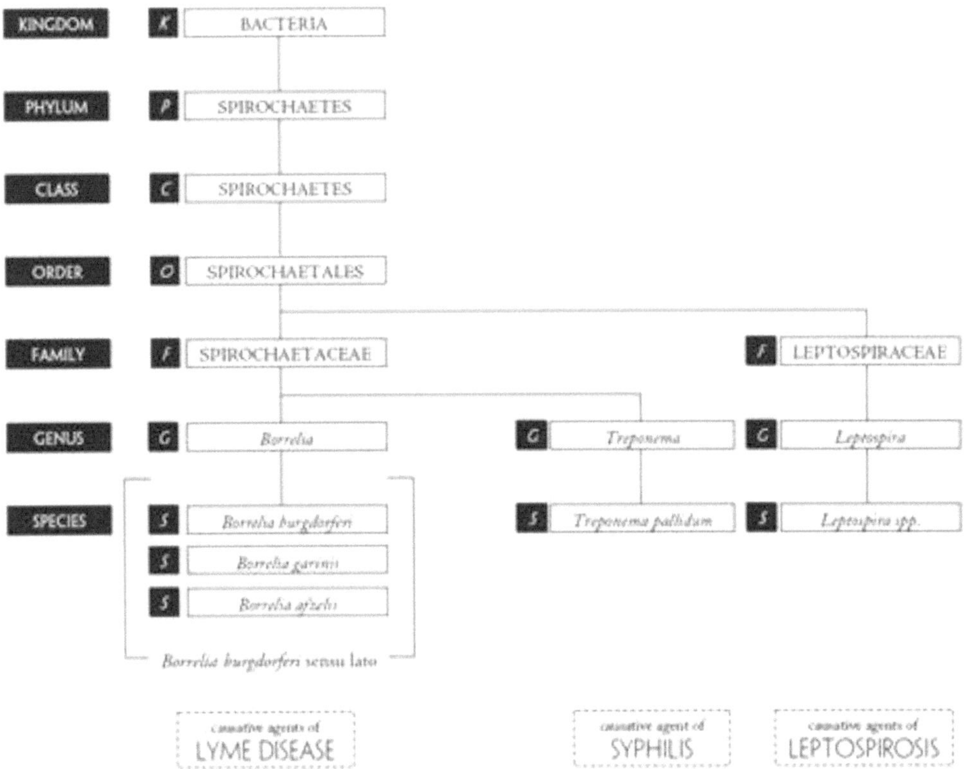

Fig. 1. Spirochaetaceae

The Spirochaetaceae family includes the genus *Treponema* and the genus *Borrelia* . *Treponema pallidum* is the causative agent of the sexually-transmitted disease syphilis.

The three members of the *Borrelia* genus *Borrelia burgdorferi* sensu stricto, *Borrelia garinii* , and *Borrelia afzelii* are collectively known as *Borrelia burgdorferi* sensu lato, and are the causative agents of Lyme disease.

1.2 Structure and morphology

Borrelia cells average 0.2 to 0.5 μm by 4 to 18 μm, and have fewer coils than *Leptospira*. The periplasmic flagella originate from either end of the spirochete (where they are anchored to the cytoplasmic membrane) and wind around the protoplasmic cylinder, imparting both motility *and* shape to the organism—in contrast to other bacteria, in which the peptidoglycan layer determines the shape.

The role of flagella in imparting *Borrelia* 's helical shape was established by inactivation of the *flaB* gene, which encodes the major flagellar filament protein, FlaB. This produced bacteria that lacked periplasmic flagella, were non-motile and rod-shaped.

Whereas the motility of externally-flagellated bacteria is hindered in viscous substances, that of spirochetes is enhanced, and about 6% of the chromosomal genome encodes proteins involved in motility and chemotaxis.

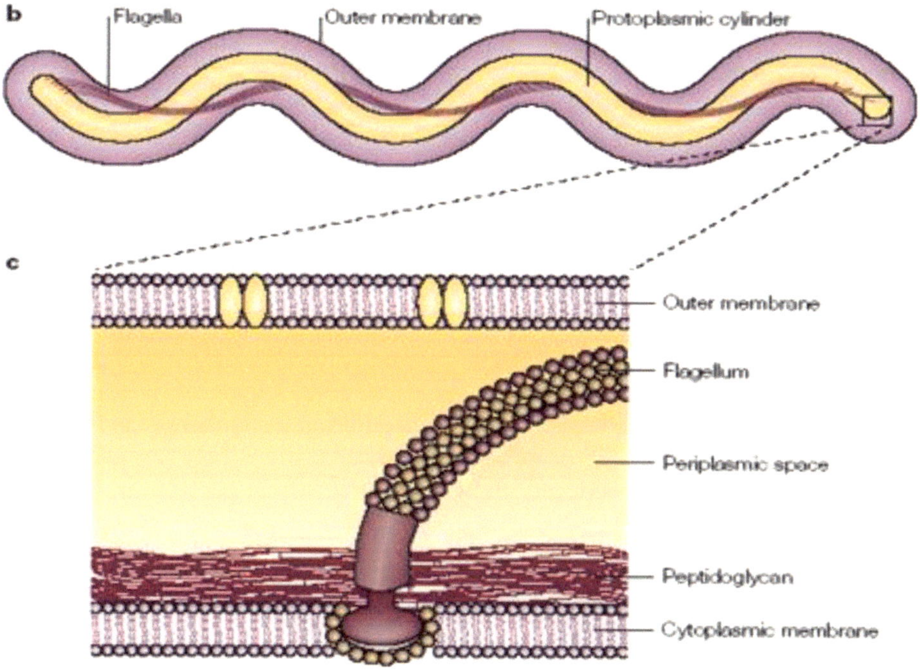
b
Flagella
Outer membrane
Protoplasmic cylinder
c
Outer membrane
Flagellum
Periplasmic space
Peptidoglycan
Cytoplasmic membrane

Fig. 2.

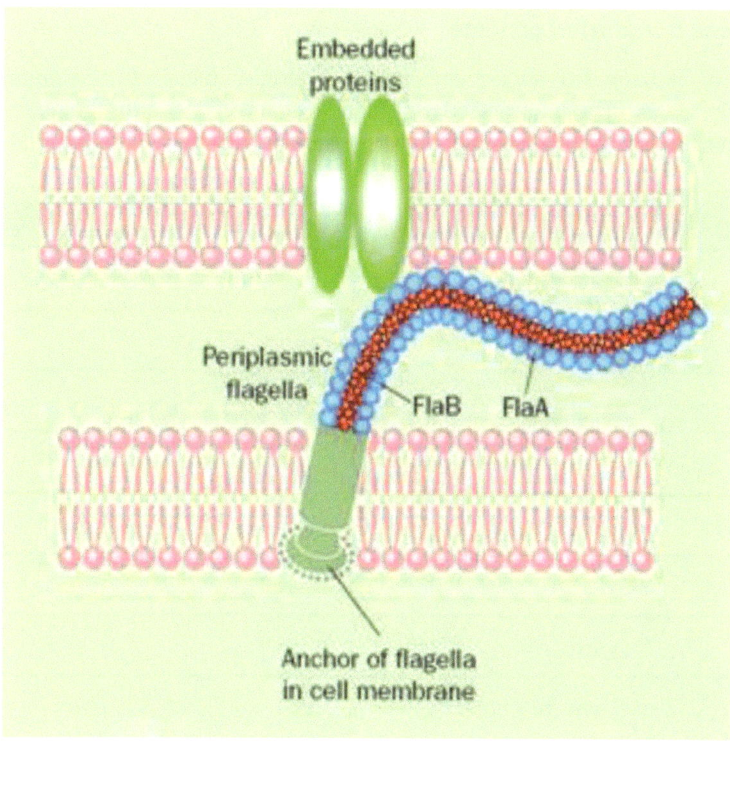
Embedded proteins
Periplasmic flagella
FlaB
FlaA
Anchor of flagella in cell membrane

Fig. 3.

1.3 Genome organization of *Borrelia burgdorferi*

All members of the *Borrelia* genus that have been examined harbor a linear chromosome that is about 900 kbp in length as well as a plethora of both linear and circular plasmids in the 5-220 kbp size range. Genome sequences have been determined for *B. burgdorferi, B. garinii, B. afzelii, B. duttonii* and *B. recurrentis*. The chromosomes, which carry the vast majority of the housekeeping genes, appear to be very constant in gene content and organization across the genus. The content of the plasmids, which carry most of the genes that encode the differentially-expressed surface proteins that interact with *Borrelia's* arthropod and vertebrate hosts, are much more variable. *B. burgdorferi* strain B31, the *B. burgdorferi* type strain, has been studied in the most detail and harbors twelve linear and nine circular plasmids that comprise about 612 kbp. The plasmids are unusual, as compared to most bacterial plasmids, in that they contain many paralogous sequences, a large number of pseudogenes and, in some cases, essential genes. In addition, a number of the plasmids have features suggesting that they are prophages. Some correlations between genome content and pathogenicity have been deduced and comparative whole genome analyses promise future progress in this arena.

The highly unusual segmented genomes of *Borrelia* species can contain over 20 utonomously replicating DNA molecules. Many of the molecules, including the chromosome, are linear with covalently closed hairpin ends.

2. Molecular biology

2.1 The *Borrelia burgdorferi* genome

The genome of *Borrelia burgdorferi* consists of a single linear chromosome and several plasmids, both linear and circular. To date—as of January 2005—only the genome of *Borrelia burgdorferi* sensu stricto B31 strain has been fully sequenced.

Distribution of cellular functions of *E. coli* and *B. burgdorferi* genes		[1]
Category	*B. burgdorferi* genes (%)	
Intermediary metabolism	4.9%	
Biosynthesis of small molecules	3.1%	
Macromolecule metabolism	22.2%	
Cell Structure	37.0%	
Cellular processes	7.4%	
Other functions	5.6%	
Unknown functions	19.8%	

Table 1.

2.2 Chromosomal genome

B. burgdorferi contains a single linear chromosome of approximately 900 kb, and about 90% of it is comprised of coding sequences. Most of the genes encoded by the chromosomal genome are homologous to genes of known function.

2.3 Extra-chromosomal genome

The extra-chromosomal genome of *B. burgdorferi* B31 consists of 12 linear plasmids and nine circular plasmids that total 610 kb in size.

2.3.1 Linear plasmids

There are two linear plasmids in *B. burgdorferi* that are absolutely necessary for persistent infection of a mammalian host. These plasmids, known as lp25 and lp28-1, are relatively unstable in culture, and are commonly lost after a few generations of *in vitro* growth. Bacteria that have lost either of these two plasmids remain capable of *in vitro* growth, but lose their ability to cause persistent infection even in immunocompromised mice. The lp25 plasmid contains a gene, *pncA*, which encodes a nicotinamidase whose function is most likely the biosynthesis of NAD; by all appearances its activity is dispensable growth *in vitro* , but crucial for growth within a host. Transforming the lp25- spirochetes with *pncA* on a shuttle vector replaces the requirement of lp25 *in vivo*. Likewise, reintroduction of the entire lp25 plasmid (by transformation) into lp25- spirochetes successfully rescues infectivity. [2]

2.3.2 Circular plasmids

An unusual feature of *B. burgdorferi* is a series of related 32-kb circular plasmids, termed cp32s. These have been found to be prophage genomes, and it is believed that they play a role in the horizontal transfer of DNA among spirochetes that share a common geographical and ecological niche. [3, 4]

2.3.3 OuterSurface Proteins (Osps)

The Outer Surface Proteins (Osps) of *B. burgdorferi* are lipoproteins that play an important role in interacting with interstitial and cellular components of insect and mammalian hosts. OspA, the most studied of the Osps, is expressed on spirochetes in unfed nymphs and adult ticks, as well as in culture. OspA mediates adherence to the cells of the tick midgut, which presumably allows spirochetes to avoid endocytosis by tick gut cells during digestion of the blood meal. The ability of *Borrelia* to regulate expression of OspA indicates that it also plays a role in detachment from the midgut, which allows the bacteria to enter the mammalian host when the tick takes a second bloodmeal.

During tick feeding, *Borrelia* in the midgut upregulate expression of another outer surface protein, OspC, and begin to move toward the salivary glands. This evident correlation suggests that OspC might play a role in transmission. Once it has entered the mammalian host, *Borrelia* downregulates OspA and exhibits variable OspC upregulation patterns. Although *B. burgdorferi* possesses only one copy of the *ospC* gene, sequences vary significantly from one strain to the next, which accounts for the observed antigenic variation between OspC proteins. The host immune system plays an important role in selecting for certain strains by eliminating the immunodominant ones.

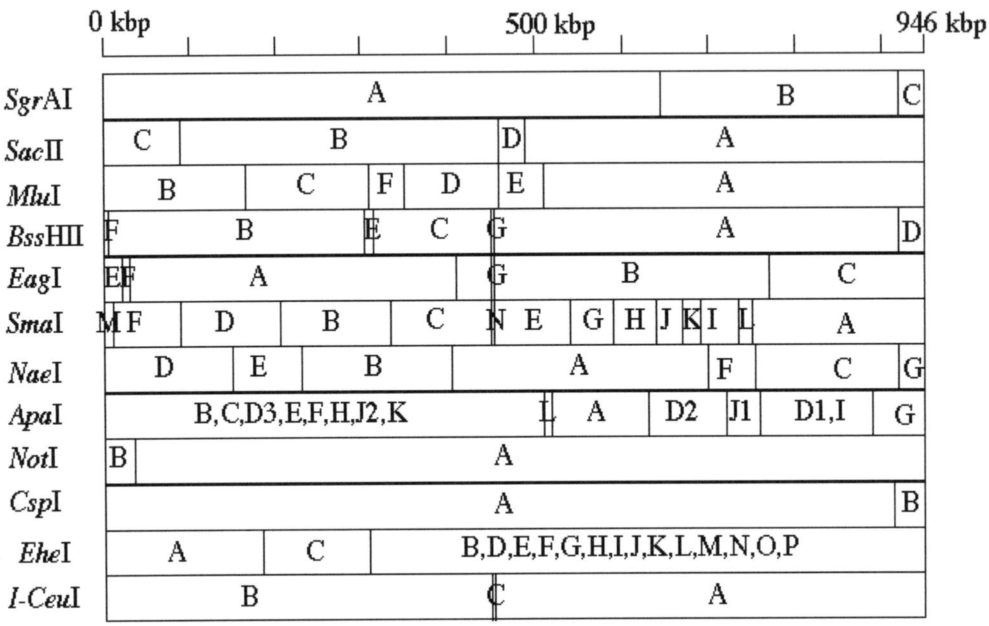

Physical map of the linear chromosome of *Borrelia burgdorferi 212*

Fig. 4.

3. Genome features in *Borrelia burgdorferi*

Chromosome 910,725 bp (28.6% G+C)

Coding sequences (93%)

RNAs (0.7%)

Intergenic sequence (6.3%)

853 coding sequences
500 (59%) with identified database match
104 (12%) match hypothetical proteins
249 (29%) with no database match

Plasmids

cp9 9,386 bp (23.6% GC)
cp26 26,497 bp (26.3% GC)

lp17 16,828 bp (23.1% GC)
lp25 24,182 bp (23.3% GC)
lp28-1 26,926 bp (32.3% GC)
lp28-2 29,771 bp (31.5% GC)
lp28-3 28,605 bp (25.1% GC)
lp28-4 27,329 bp (24.4% GC)
lp36 36,834 bp (26.8% GC)
lp38 38,853 bp (26.1% GC)
lp54 53,590 bp (28.1% GC)
Coding sequences (71%)
Intergenic sequence (29%)
430 coding sequences
70 (16%) with identified database match
110 (26%) match hypothetical proteins
250 (58%) with no database match

Ribosomal RNA Chromosome coordinates

16S 444581–446118
23S 438590–441508
5S 438446–438557
23S 435334–438267
5S 435201–435312

Stable RNA

tmRNA 46973–47335
mpB 750816–751175

Transfer RNA

34 species (8 clusters,14 single genes)

*The telomeric sequences of the nine linear plasmids assembled as part of this study were not determined; estimation of the number of missing terminal nucleotides by restriction analysis suggests that less than 1,200 bp is missing in all cases. Comparisons with previously determined sequences of lp 16.9 and one terminus of lp28-1 indicate that 25, 60 and 1,200 bp are missing, respectively.

Chromosomally-encoded genes

- rRNA sequences
- fla sequences
- hbb sequences
- fesmid sequences

3.1 *Borrelia burgdorferi* rRNA sequences

Genbank mnemomic	Accession number	Description	Strain	Date of entry	Size
Gb_ba:Bbrnaopr	U03396	*alaT* (Ala-tRNA), *ileT* (Ile-tRNA), *rrs* (16S rRNA), *rrlA* & *rrlB* (23S rRNA) *rrfA* & *rrfB* (5S rRNA)	B31	10/93	11955bp
Gb_ba:Bbu44938	U44938	*rrs* (16S rRNA)	5MT	5/96	1,533bp
Gb_ba:Bor16rg	L39080	*rrs* (16S rRNA)	9MT	3/95	1,533bp
Gb_ba:Bbu44939	U44939	*rrs* (16S rRNA)	917Y	5/96	1,533bp
Gb_ba:Bb16s297	X85204	*rrs* (16S rRNA)	297	5/95	1,488bp
Gb_ba:Borrrd	L36160	*rrs* (16S rRNA)	934U	9/94	1,536bp
Gb_ba:Bor16rga	L39081	*rrs* (16S rRNA)	935T	3/95	1,542bp
Gb_ba:Borrrdq	M64309	*rrs* (16S rRNA)	1352	4/92	1,481bp
Gb_ba:Borrrd	M64310	*rrs* (16S rRNA)	20004	4/92	1,480bp
Gb_ba:Bb16srrna	X57404	*rrs* (16S rRNA)	B31	3/92	1,465bp
Gb_ba:Borssrna	M59293	*rrs* (16S rRNA)	B31	4/92	1,480bp
Gb_ba:Borrnaca	M89935	*rrs* (16S rRNA)	CA2-87	1/93	1,291bp
Gb_ba:Bb16sdk7	X85195	*rrs* (16S rRNA)	DK7	5/95	1,488bp
Gb_ba:Bb16sdk29	X85202	*rrs* (16S rRNA)	DK29	5/95	1,488bp
Gb_ba:Bb16sdunk	X85201	*rrs* (16S rRNA)	DUNKIRK	5/95	1,488bp
Gb_ba:Bbu28501	U28501	*rrs* (16S rRNA)	ESP-1	7/95	1,488bp
Gb_ba:Borrr16sa	M60967	*rrs* (16S rRNA)	G2	4/92	1,483bp
Gb_ba:Borrnail	M89936	*rrs* (16S rRNA)	Illinois 1	1/93	1,291bp
Gb_ba:Bb16skipp	X85196	*rrs* (16S rRNA)	KIPP	5/95	1,488bp
Gb_ba:Bb16slipz	X85203	*rrs* (16S rRNA)	LIPITZ	5/95	1,488bp
Gb_ba:Borrr16sc	M60969	*rrs* (16S rRNA)	Sh-2-82	4/92	1,476bp
Gb_ba:Borrnavs	M89938	*rrs* (16S rRNA)	VS219	1/93	1,350bp
Gb_ba:Borrgda	L40596	*rrs* (16S rRNA)		3/95	1,492bp

Genbank mnemomic	Accession number	Description	Strain	Date of entry	Size
Gb_ba:Borrg16s	M88329	*rrs* (16S rRNA)		11/93	1,537bp
Gb_ba:Bor23srrna	M93664	*rr1* (23S rRNA)	212	6/92	398bp
Gb_ba:Bb23s5s	X85745	*rrl rrs* (23S & 5S rRNA)	B31	7/95	2,093bp
Gb_ba:Borrg23s	M88330	*rr1* (23S rRNA)		1/93	2,926bp
Gb_ba:Bb523srr	X57791	*rrf* (5S) and *rrl* (23S rRNA genes).		6/93	616bp
Gb_ba:Borburssp	L30121	internal transcribed spacer	212	7/94	253bp
Gb_ba:Borburs2sp	L30127	internal transcribed spacer	B31	7/94	254bp
Gb_ba:Borburg7sp	L30123	internal transcribed spacer	CA2	7/94	255bp

Table 2.

3.2 *Borrelia burgdorferi* fla sequences

Genbank mnemomic	Accession number	Description	Strain	Date of entry	Size
Gb_ba:Borflass	L29234	*fla* (flagellin)	212	7/94	193bp
Gb_ba:Bbfaa	X16833	*fla* flagellum-associated 41kD antigen (flagellin)	B31	9/93	1,435bp
Gb_ba:Bbfla2	X15661	*fla* (flagellin)	B31	2/94	1,011bp
Gb_ba:Borflab31a	L29200	*fla* (flagellin)	B31	7/94	193bp
Gb_ba:Borflag	M34710	*fla* (flagellin)	B31	5/95	684bp
Gb_ba:Bbbop41	X69607	*fla* flagellum-associated 41kD antigen (flagellin)	BO	5/94	1,008bp
Gb_ba:Bbgehofla	X56334	*fla* (flagellin)	GeHo	4/93	1,426bp
Gb_ba:Bbfla	X15660	*fla* (flagellin)	GeHo	2/94	1,011bp

Genbank mnemomic	Accession number	Description	Strain	Date of entry	Size
Gb_ba:Bbflagen	X75200	*fla* (flagellin)	HB19	8/95	1,117bp
Gb_ba:Bbflagen	X75200	*fla* (flagellin)	HB19	12/93	1,117bp
Gb_ba:Bbhep41	X69609	*fla* flagellum-associated 41kD antigen (flagellin)	HE	5/94	1,011bp
Gb_ba:Bbkap41	X69611	*fla* flagellum-associated 41kD antigen (flagellin)	KA	5/94	1,008bp
Gb_ba:Bor2fla	L42881	*fla* (flagellin)	KL10	6/95	1,011bp
Gb_ba:Bor1fla	L42876	*fla* (flagellin)	NBS1ab	6/95	1,011bp
Gb_ba:Borflac	M67458	*fla* (flagellin)	PSto	5/92	226bp
Gb_ba:Bbtrop41	X69614	*fla* flagellum-associated 41kD antigen (flagellin)	TRO	5/94	1,011bp

Table 3.

3.3 *Borrelia burgdorferi hbb* sequences

Genbank mnemomic	Accession number	Description	Strain	Date of entry	Size
Gb_ba:Bbu48650	U48650	*hbb* (Histone like protein HBbu)	A44S	4/96	327bp
Gb_ba:Bbu48648	U48648	*hbb* (Histone like protein HBbu)	B31	4/96	327bp
Gb_ba:Bbu48652	U48652	*hbb* (Histone like protein HBbu)	IP1	4/96	327bp
Gb_ba:Bbu48653	U48653	*hbb* (Histone like protein HBbu)	IP2	4/96	327bp
Gb_ba:Bbu48648	U48648	*hbb* (Histone like protein HBbu)	B31	4/96	327bp
Gb_ba:Bbu48649	U48649	*hbb* (Histone like protein HBbu)	NY13-87	4/96	327bp
Gb_ba:Bbu48654	U48654	*hbb* (Histone like protein HBbu)	IP3	4/96	327bp
Gb_ba:Bbu35673	U35673	*hbb* (Histone like protein HBbu)	Sh-2-82	10/95	3,399bp

Table 4.

3.4 *Borrelia burgdorferi* fesmid sequences

Genbank mnemomic	Accession number	Description	Strain	Date of entry	Size
Gb_ba:Bbu43739	U43739	Genes noted below	B31	1/96	34,817bp

Table 5.

orf38 (open reading frame);
orf37 (open reading frame);
orf36 (open reading frame);
ylxH (putative ATP-binding protein);
flhF (flagella asociated putative GTP-binding protein protein);
flhA (flagellar protein required for flagellar formation);
flhB (flagellar protein required for flagellar formation);
fliR (flagellar protein required for flagellar formation);
fliQ (flagellar protein required for flagellar formation);
fliP (flagellar protein required for flagellar formation);
fliZ (flagellar protein required for flagellar formation);
fliN (flagellar switch protein);
fliM (flagellar switch protein);
orf25 (open reading frame);
motB (flagellar motor rotation protein B);
motA (flagellar motor rotation protein A);
flgE (flagellar hook protein);
ylxG (flagellar synthesis);
orf20 (open reading frame);
orf19 (open reading frame);
orf18 (open reading frame);
fliI (flagellar synthesis);
fliH (flagellar synthesis);
fliG (flagellar switch protein);
fliF (flagella basal-body M ring protein);
fliE (flagella basal-body protein);
flgC (flagella associated rod protein);
flgB (flagella associated rod protein);
hslU heat shock protein);
hslV (heat shock protein);
smg (?);
orf7 (open reading frame);
ftsZ (cell division protein);
ftsA (cell division protein);
divIB (cell division protein);
ftsW (cell division protein);
mraY (phosphotransferase);
murF (pentapeptide presynthetase)

3.5 *Borrelia burgdorferi* chromosomal sequences (Except rrn & fla genes)

Genbank mnemomic	Accession number	Description	Strain	Date of entry	Size
Gb_ba:Borp39ant	L24194	*bmpA bmpB* (immunodo-minant antigen P39 gene)	Sh-2-82	7/94	2,304bp
Gb_ba:Borbmpa	L35050	*bmpA bmpB* (membrane lipoproteins A & B	212	12/94	904bp
Gb_ba:Borbmpc	L34547	*bmpC* (membrane lipoprotein C)	297	11/94	1,293bp
Gb_ba:Bbu35450	L34547	*bmpD* (membrane lipoprotein D)	297	4/96	1,525bp
Gb_ba:Bbcheagen	X91907	*cheA1* (histidine kinase)	212	9/95	332bp
Gb_ba:Bbu28962	U28962	*cheA1* (histidine kinase)	CT-1	6/95	2,491bp
Gb_ba:Borchea	L39965	*cheA2* (histidine kinase)	B31	8/95	2,410bp
Gb_ba: Bbu34384	U34384	*cheW* (Positive regulator of CheA activity)	CT-1	9/95	660bp
Gb_ba:Bbu04527	U04527	*dnaA* (DNA replication initiatior), *dnaN* (DNA polymerase III beta subunit),*gyrB* (DNA gyrase B subunit), *rpmH* (ribosomal pro-tein L34) and *rnpA* (ribonuclease P protein component)	212	2/94	4943bp
Gb_ba:Borgrpepls	M96847	*dnaJ dnaK*and *grpE* (heat shock proteins)		2/93	3913bp
Gb_ba:Bordnaj	M97914	*dnaJ*(heat-shock protein)	CA12	12/92	1,094bp
Gb_ba:Borhsp70a	M97912	*dnaK* (70 kDa heat shock protein)	CA12	10/92	1,928bp
Gb_ba:S42385	S42385	*dnaK* (70 kDa heat shock protein)	CA12	10/92	1,911bp
Gb_ba:Bbhspro	X67646	*dnaK* (70 kDa heat-shock protein)	ZS7	8/92	2,116bp
Gb_ba:Bbu12870	U12870	*flgE* (flagellar hook polypeptide)	N40	4/95	1,552bp
Gb_ba:Bbu19712	U19712	*flgE* (flagellar hook polypeptide)	B31	1/95	571bp
Gb_ba:Borflge	L43849	*flgE* (flagellar hook polypeptide)	HB19	8/95	1499bp
Gb_ba:Borflif	L40501	*fliF* (Flagellar MS-ring protein)	212	2/96	1717bp
Gb_ba:BBU09711	U09711	*fliG* (Flagellar switch protein)	212	7/95	1035bp
Gb_ba:Borflih	L40502	*fliH* (export of flagellar proteins?)	212	1/96	921 bp
Gb_ba:Borflii	L43325	*fliI* (export of flagellar proteins?)	212	1/96	1311 bp

Genbank mnemomic	Accession number	Description	Strain	Date of entry	Size
Gb_ba:Bbftszg	Z12164	*ftsZ* (cell division protein)	212	5/94	261bp
Gb_ba:Bbu28760	U28760	*gapDH* (glyceraldehyde-3-phosphate dehydro-genase); *pgk* phosphogly-cerate kinase; *tpi* triose-phosphate isomerase	B31	6/95	798bp
Gb_ba:Bbgidag	Z12160	*gidA* (glucose inhibited division protein)	212	5/94	196bp
Gb_ba:Bbhsp60	X65139	*groEL*(common antigen)	ZS7	5/92	1,931bp
Gb_ba:Bbgyrag	Z12165	*gyrA* (DNA gyrase subunit A)	212	5/94	289bp
Gb_ba:Bbgyrbg	Z12166	*gyrB*(DNA gyrase subunit B)	212	5/94	253bp
Gb_ba:Borhtpg	L32145	*htpG* (C62.5 heat shock protein)	212	12/94	236bp
Gb_ba:Borlonaa	L77216	*lon* ATP-dependent protease	B31	4/96	2,946bp
Gb_ba:Bormetg	L32146	*metG* (methionyl tRNA synthetase)	212	12/94	346bp
Gb_ba:Borplsctop	L32861	*parE* (topoisomerase IV, B subunit), *plsC* (1-acyl-sn-glycerol-3-phosphate acetyltransferase)	212	5/94	677bp
Gb_ba:Bbysc1	X78708	*pep* APE1 (aminopepti-dase 1 homologue)	ZS7	4/94	1,776bp
Gb_ba:Borpgktpi	L32595	*pgk* (phosphoglycerate kinase), *tpi* (triose-phosphate isomerase)	212	5/94	370bp
Gb_ba:Borpthh	L32144	*pth* (peptidyl-tRNA hydrolase)	212	4/94	910bp
Gb_ba:Bbu23457	U23457	*recA* General recombi-nation & DNA repair	Sh-2-82	4/96	2,025bp
Gb_ba:Borrho	L07656	*rho* (Rho protein)	Sh-2-82	9/93	1,499bp
Gb_ba:Borrpob	L48488	*rpoB rpoC* (RNA polymerase, beta & beta prime subunits)	B31	11/95	3,682bp
Gb_ba:Borrhoa	L46347	*rho* (Rho protein)	212	8/95	571bp
Gb_ba:Bbu35673	U35673	*rpsT* (30S ribosomal protein S20)	Sh-2-82	10/95	3,399bp
Gb_ba:Bbrnasep	U17591	*rpoD* (primary sigma factor)	B31	12/94	4,165bp
Gb_ba:Bortufz	L23125	*tuf* (elongation factor EF-Tu)	B31	8/93	1,230bp

Table 6.

3.6 *Borrelia burgdorferi* chromosomal sequences (Antigens and proteins of unknown function)

Genbank mnemomic	Accession number	Description	Strain	Date of entry	Size
Gb_ba:Bororf	L32797	p21 (21 kDa protein)		5/95	1,152bp
Gb_ba:Borunk	L31615	p21A (21 kD protein)	297	8/94	700bp
Gb_ba:Bor22kdant	M90084	p22 (22 kD antigen)	B31	10/93	795bp
Gb_ba:Borp22x	L22530	p22X (22 kD outer surface lipoprotein)	N40	8/94	585bp
Gb_ba:Borp23a	L31616	p23 (23kD protein)	297	8/94	686bp
Gb_ba:Bbhypp	X63898	p38 (38 kD ATP-binding protein)	GeHo	2/92	1,435bp
Gb_ba:Bdna66kd	X87725	p66 (66 kD protein)	B31	6/95	2,180bp
Gb_ba:Borlyme	L32596	p66 (66 kD protein)	212	6/92	240bp
Gb_ba:Bbp831001	X81514	p93/p100 (93 kD protein)	297	7/95	287bp
Gb_ba:Bbbop93	X69601	p93 (93 kD protein)	BO	12/93	1,991bp
Gb_ba:Bbp97	X77749	p97 (97 kD protein)	GOE2	6/95	2,082bp
Gb_ba:Bbp831002	X81520	p93/p100 (93 kD protein)	pacificus	7/95	269bp
Gb_ba:Bbp83100	X81357	p83/p100 (100 kD protein)	PBre	4/96	287bp
Gb_ba:Bbp831003	X81528	p93/p100 (93 kD protein)	PKa2	7/95	287bp
Gb_ba:Bbp831004	X81531	p93/p100 (93 kD protein)	T255	7/95	287bp
Gb_ba:Bbtrop93	X69604	p93 (93 kD protein)	TRO	12/93	2,081bp
Gb_ba:Borsurant	L36037	surface antigen	Dk1	9/94	185bp
Gb_ba:Bbla7	X70826	LA7 (21 kD lipoprotein)	ZS7	11/93	821bp
Gb_ba:	X91965	*abp* (probable ATP binding protein)	212	9/95	285bp
Gb_ba:Boraaa	M60802	immunogen gene		12/92	2,258bp
Gb_ba:Bbu18292	U18292	"bbk2.10 gene"	297	7/95	1,799bp
Gb_ba:Bbu19105	U19105	"bbk2.10 gene"	N40	7/95	832bp
Gb_ba:Borlyme	L32596	PCR target	212	8/94	240bp

Genbank mnemomic	Accession number	Description	Strain	Date of entry	Size
Gb_ba:Borseqa	M58429	PCR target		3/91	379bp
Gb_ba:Borseqc	M58431	PCR target		3/91	1725bp
Gb_ba:Borseqd	M58432	PCR target		3/91	381bp
Gb_ba:Borseqe	M58433	PCR target		3/91	379bp
Gb_ba:Bbu35673	U35673	*orfH, orfR and hbbU* (putative proteins)	Sh-2-82	10/95	3,399bp

Table 7.

Plasmid-encoded genes

- ospA genes
- ospB genes
- ospC genes
- ospD genes

3.7 *Borrelia burgdorferi* Plasmid-encoded sequences (Except ospA, ospB, ospC & ospD)

Genbank mnemomic	Accession number	Description	Plasmid	Strain	Date of entry	Size
Gb_ba: Borgmpguaa	L25883	*guaA* (GMP synthetase)	26 kb cp	CA-11.2A	11/94	1,599bp
Gb_ba:Bbu13372	U13372	*guaB* (IMP dehydrogenase)	26 kb cp	CA-11.2A	11/94	1,212bp
Gb_ba:Borospea	L13924	*ospE* (outer surface protein E)	45kb lp	N40	3/94	644bp
Gb_ba:Borospfa	L13925	*ospF* (outer surface protein F)	45kb lp	N40	3/94	785bp
Gb_ba:Bbu19754	U19754	*ospF* (outer surface protein F)	45kb lp	297	7/95	690bp
Gb_ba:Bbospg	X82409	*ospG* & *bapA* (outer surface protein G & associated protein A)	48b lp	ZS7	11/95	1524bp
Gb_ba:Bbu22451	U22451	p12 (12kDa lipoprotein)	49kb lp	B31	3/95	285bp
Gb_ba: Borexpprtn	L16625	p20 (exported neuro-toxin-like protein)	9kb cp	B31	8/94	720bp
Gb_ba:S66708	S66708	PCR target sequence	30kb cp	B31	11/95	416bp

Genbank mnemomic	Accession number	Description	Plasmid	Strain	Date of entry	Size
Gb_ba:Bors1a	L34016	S1 antigen	49kb lp	N40	11/95	1,421bp
Gb_ba:Bors2a	L34016	S2 antigen	49kb lp	N40	11/95	837bp
Gb_ba: Bbptl4916	X53311	telomeres pTL16 and pTL49	16kb lp & 49kb lp		2/93	238bp
Gb_ba:Bbptr16	X53312	telomere pTR16	16 kb lp		2/93	191bp
Gb_ba:S65114	S65114	left terminal repeat, telomeric fragment	lp		7/92	38bp
Gb_ba:	X87127	repeated DNA element	30.5kb cp		4/96	5,500bp

Table 8.

3.8 *Borrelia burgdorferi* ospA sequences

Genbank mnemomic	Accession number	Description	Strain	Date of entry	Size
Gb_ba:Bb297ospa	X85442	*ospA* (outer surface protein A)	297	8/95	822bp
Gb_ba:Borospad	L23138	*ospA ospB* (outer surface proteins A & B)	19535NY2	8/94	1,653bp
Gb_ba:Borospah	L23141	*ospA ospB* (outer surface proteins A & B)	21343WI	8/94	1,653bp
Gb_ba:Borospac	L23137	*ospA ospB* (outer surface proteins A & B)	27985CT2	6/94	1,653bp
Gb_ba:Borospaf	L23140	*ospA ospB* (outer surface proteins A & B)	41552MA	8/94	1,653bp
Gb_ba:Borospae	L23139	*ospA ospB* (outer surface proteins A & B)	42373NY3	8/94	1,653bp
Gb_ba:Borospaa	L23136	*ospA ospB* (outer surface proteins A & B)	B19CT1	6/94	1,653bp
Gb_ba:Bbospab	X14407	*ospA ospB* (outer surface proteins A & B)	B31	9/94	1,915bp
Gb_ba:Boropsab	L19701	*ospA ospB* (outer surface proteins A & B)	B31	6/93	1,916b

Genbank mnemomic	Accession number	Description	Strain	Date of entry	Size
Gb_ba:Borospai	L23142	*ospA ospB* (outer surface proteins A & B)	CA3	8/94	1,653bp
Gb_ba:Borospaj	L23143	*ospA ospB* (outer surface proteins A & B)	CA7	8/94	1,653bp
Gb_ba:Borospak	L23144	*ospA ospB* (outer surface proteins A & B)	CA8	8/94	1,653bp
Gb_ba:Bbdk6ospa	X83622	*ospA* (outer surface protein A)	DK6	1/95	822bp
Gb_ba:Bbpospa	X63412	*ospA* (outer surface protein A)	DK29	1/94	825bp
Gb_ba:Bormajospr	L19702	*ospA* (outer surface protein A)	G2	6/93	2,123bp
Gb_ba:Bbaspa	X60300	*ospA* (outer surface protein A)	Goe2	12/92	1,361bp
Gb_ba:Borospaa	L23136	*ospA ospB* (outer surface proteins A & B)	HB19CT1	6/94	1,653bp
Gb_ba:Bbospa3	X65600	*ospA* (outer surface protein A)	HE	1/94	822bp
Gb_ba:Bbu33179	U33179	*ospA* (outer surface protein A)	HT29	9/95	270bp
Gb_ba:Bbopsaa	X70365	*ospA* (outer surface protein A)	IP3	5/94	822bp
Gb_ba:Bbka0spa	X69606	*ospA* (outer surface protein A)	KA	5/94	822bp
Gb_ba:Bbospcmul	X84779	*ospA* (outer surface protein A)	MUL	5/95	534bp
Gb_ba:Borfra	L38657	*ospA* (outer surface protein A)	N3	1/95	822bp
Gb_ba:Borospa	M57248	*ospA* (outer surface protein A)	N40	11/91	819bp
Gb_ba:Bbdnaospa	X85739	*ospA* (outer surface protein A)	PBre	9/95	822bp
Gb_ba:Bbpheiosp	X80251	*ospA* (outer surface protein A)	PHei	9/95	822bp
Gb_ba:Bbpkaospa	X80182	*ospA* (outer surface protein A)	PKa	9/95	822bp
Gb_ba:Bbpwud1	X80184	*ospA* (outer surface protein A)	PWud1	9/95	822bp
Gb_ba:Bbpwudi	X68540	*ospA* (outer surface protein A)	PWudI	3/93	333bp
Gb_ba:Bbpwudl6	X80185	*ospA* (outer surface protein A)	PWud1/6	9/95	822bp
Gb_ba:Bbpwudll	X80253	*ospA* (outer surface protein A)	PWud11	9/95	825bp

Genbank mnemomic	Accession number	Description	Strain	Date of entry	Size
Gb_ba:Bbpwudii	X68539	*ospA* (outer surface protein A)	PWudII	3/93	333bp
Gb_ba:Bor90ospa	L42873	*ospA* (outer surface protein A)	SIMON	6/95	582bp
Gb_ba:Bbt25ospa	X85443	*ospA* (outer surface protein A)	T255	9/95	822bp
Gb_ba:Borospaab	D29660	*ospA* (outer surface protein A)	tick isolate	4/95	911bp
Gb_ba:Bbospa1	X65598	*ospA* (outer surface protein A)	TRO	1/94	822bp
Gb_ba:Bbospa	X16467	*ospA* (outer surface protein A)	ZS7	9/93	942bp
Gb_ba:A22442	A22442	*ospA* (outer surface protein A)	ZS7	12/94	822bp
Gb_ba:Bbosproa	X66065	*ospA* (outer surface protein A)	ZQ1	7/93	825bp
Gb_ba:A24006	A24006	*ospA* (outer surface protein A)	ZQ1	2/95	825bp
Gb_ba:A04009	A04009	*ospA ospB* (outer surface proteins A & B)		4/93	1,915bp

Table 9.

3.9 *Borrelia burgdorferi* ospB sequences

Genbank mnemomic	Accession number	Description	Strain	Date of entry	Size
Gb_ba:Borospad	L23138	*ospA ospB* (outer surface proteins A & B)	19535NY2	8/94	1,653bp
Gb_ba:Borospah	L23141	*ospA ospB* (outer surface proteins A & B)	21343WI	8/94	1,653bp
Gb_ba:Borospac	L23137	*ospA ospB* (outer surface proteins A & B)	27985CT2	6/94	1,653bp
Gb_ba:Borospaf	L23140	*ospA ospB* (outer surface proteins A & B)	41552MA	8/94	1,653bp
Gb_ba:Borospae	L23139	*ospA ospB* (outer surface proteins A & B)	42373NY3	8/94	1,653bp
Gb_ba:Boropsab	L19701	*ospA ospB* (outer surface proteins A & B)	B31	6/93	1,916b
Gb_ba:Bbospab	X14407	*ospA ospB* (outer surface proteins A & B)	B31	9/94	1,915bp

Genbank mnemomic	Accession number	Description	Strain	Date of entry	Size
Gb_ba:Bbospbb31	X74808	*ospB* (outer surface protein B)	B31	7/94	934bp
Gb_ba:Bbospbev	X74810	*ospB* (outer surface protein B)	B31/EVB	7/94	934bp
Gb_ba:Bbospbbp	X74809	*ospB* (outer surface protein B)	BEP4	7/94	934bp
Gb_ba:Borospai	L23142	*ospA ospB* (outer surface proteins A & B)	CA3	8/94	1,653bp
Gb_ba:Borospaj	L23143	*ospA ospB* (outer surface proteins A & B)	CA7	8/94	1,653bp
Gb_ba:Borospak	L23144	*ospA ospB* (outer surface proteins A & B)	CA8	8/94	1,653bp
Gb_ba:Borospbvr	L31399	*ospB* (outer surface protein B)	HB19	3/95	891bp
Gb_ba:Borospaa	L23136	*ospA ospB* (outer surface proteins A & B)	HB19CT1	6/94	1,653bp
Gb_ba:A04009	A04009	*ospA ospB* (outer surface proteins A & B)		4/93	1,915bp

Table 10.

3.10 *Borrelia burgdorferi* ospC sequences

Genbank mnemomic	Accession number	Description	Strain	Date of entry	Size
Gb_ba:Bbospc272	X84785	*ospC* (outer surface protein C)	272	5/95	534bp
Gb_ba:Bbu08284	U08284	*ospC* (outer surface protein C)	297	9/94	579bp
Gb_ba:Bor26ospc	L42893	*ospC* (outer surface protein C)	297	6/95	576bp
Gb_ba:Bbu01892	U01892	*ospC* (outer surface protein C)	2591	1/94	824bp
Gb_ba:Bor32ospc	L42899	*ospC* (outer surface protein C)	21347	6/95	576bp
Gb_ba:Bor30ospc	L42897	*ospC* (outer surface protein C)	26815	6/95	579bp
Gb_ba:Bor29ospc	L42896	*ospC* (outer surface protein C)	27579	6/95	573bp
Gb_ba:Bor28ospc	L42895	*ospC* (outer surface protein C)	28354	6/95	579bp
Gb_ba:Bor27ospc	L42894	*ospC* (outer surface protein C)	28691	6/95	573bp

Genbank mnemomic	Accession number	Description	Strain	Date of entry	Size
Gb_ba:Bbb31ospc	X69596	*ospC* (outer surface protein C)	B31	5/93	633bp
Gb_ba:Bbu01894	U01894	*ospC* (outer surface protein C)	B31	1/94	980bp
Gb_ba:Borospca	D49497	*ospC* (outer surface protein C)	B31	5/95	633bp
Gb_ba:Bbospcbur	X84765	*ospC* (outer surface protein C)	BUR	5/95	534bp
Gb_ba:Borospc	L25413	*ospC* (outer surface protein C)	CA-11.2A	7/94	1,150bp
Gb_ba:Bbospce	X73626	*ospC* (outer surface protein C)	DK6	2/94	609bp
Gb_ba:Bbospcd	X73625	*ospC* (outer surface protein C)	DK7	2/94	618bp
Gb_ba:Bbospcc	X73624	*ospC* (outer surface protein C)	DK26	2/94	624bp
Gb_ba:Bbospcb	X73623	*ospC* (outer surface protein C)	DK27	2/94	624bp
Gb_ba:Bbospcduk	X84778	*ospC* (outer surface protein C)	DUNKIRK	5/95	528bp
Gb_ba:Bbu04281	U04281	*ospC* (outer surface protein C)	HB19	1/95	692bp
Gb_ba:Bor20ospc	L42887	*ospC* (outer surface protein C)	Ip2	6/95	576bp
Gb_ba:Bbospckip	X84782	*ospC* (outer surface protein C)	KIPP	5/95	534bp
Gb_ba:Bbu04240	U04240	*ospC* (outer surface protein C)	N40	8/94	689bp
Gb_ba:Bbdnaospc	X83555	*ospC* (outer surface protein C)	pacificus	6/95	630bp
Gb_ba:Bbospc1	X81522	*ospC* (outer surface protein C)	PBre	6/95	636bp
Gb_ba:Bbpkaospc	X69589	*ospC* (outer surface protein C)	PKa	2/94	633bp
Gb_ba:Bbt25ospc	X69592	*ospC* (outer surface protein C)	T25	2/94	636bp
Gb_ba:Bbospc2	X81524	*ospC* (outer surface protein C)	T255	5/95	633bp
Gb_ba:Bbospctxw	X84783	*ospC* (outer surface protein C)	TXGW	5/95	531bp
Gb_ba:Bbwudospc	X69590	*ospC* (outer surface protein C)	WudI	2/94	639bp
Gb_ba:Bor40ospc	L42868	*ospC* (outer surface protein C)	ZS7	6/95	579bp

Table 11.

3.11 *Borrelia burgdorferi* ospD sequences

Genbank mnemomic	Accession number	Description	Strain	Date of entry	Size
Gb_ba:Bbu05304	U05304	*ospD* (outer surface protein D)	3028	11/94	1,012bp
Gb_ba:Bbu05305	U05305	*ospD* (outer surface protein D)	27985	11/94	1,012bp
Gb_ba:Borospd	M97452	*ospD* (outer surface protein D)	B31	2/93	1,079bp
Gb_ba:Bbu05324	U05324	*ospD* (outer surface protein D)	CA12	11/94	991bp
Gb_ba:Borospdhb	L34055	*ospD* (outer surface protein D)	HB19	6/94	1,045bp
Gb_ba:Bbu05327	U05327	*ospD* (outer surface protein D)	lp7	11/94	1,064bp

Table 12.

3.12 *Borrelia burgdorferi* fusion sequences

Genbank mnemomic	Accession number	Description	Strain	Date of entry	Size
Gb_ba:A24010	A24010	*ospA* fusion	NS1	2/95	1,020bp
Gb_ba:A24012	A24012	*ospA* fusion	NS1	2/95	1,014bp
Gb_ba:A24014	A24014	*ospA* fusion	NS1	2/95	1,017bp
Gb_ba:A24016	A24016	*ospA* fusion	NS1	2/95	1,017bp
Gb_ba:Borbb1	L31427	*phoA* fusion	297	4/95	279bp
Gb_ba:Borbb10	L31421	*phoA* fusion	297	4/95	319bp
Gb_ba:Borbb11	L31424	*phoA* fusion	297	4/95	248bp
Gb_ba:Borbb13	L31422	*phoA* fusion	297	4/95	354bp
Gb_ba:Borbb14	L31423	*phoA* fusion	297	4/95	361bp
Gb_ba:Borbb16	L31425	*phoA* fusion	297	4/95	135bp
Gb_ba:Borbb17	L31426	*phoA* fusion	297	4/95	615bp
Gb_ba:Borbb4	L31417	*phoA* fusion	297	4/95	294bp
Gb_ba:Borbb4a	L31419	*phoA* fusion	297.	4/95	221bp
Gb_ba:Borbb5	L31418	*phoA* fusion	297	4/95	341bp
Gb_ba:Borbb9	L31420	*phoA* fusion	297	4/95	233bp

Table 13.

3.13 *Borrelia burgdorferi* promoter sequences

Genbank mnemomic	Accession number	Description	Strain	Date of entry	Size
Gb_ba:Borproma	M28680	promoter	B31	6/90	194bp
Gb_ba:Borpromb	M28681	promoter	B31	6/90	203bp
Gb_ba:Borpromc	M28682	promoter	B31	6/90	78bp

Table 14.

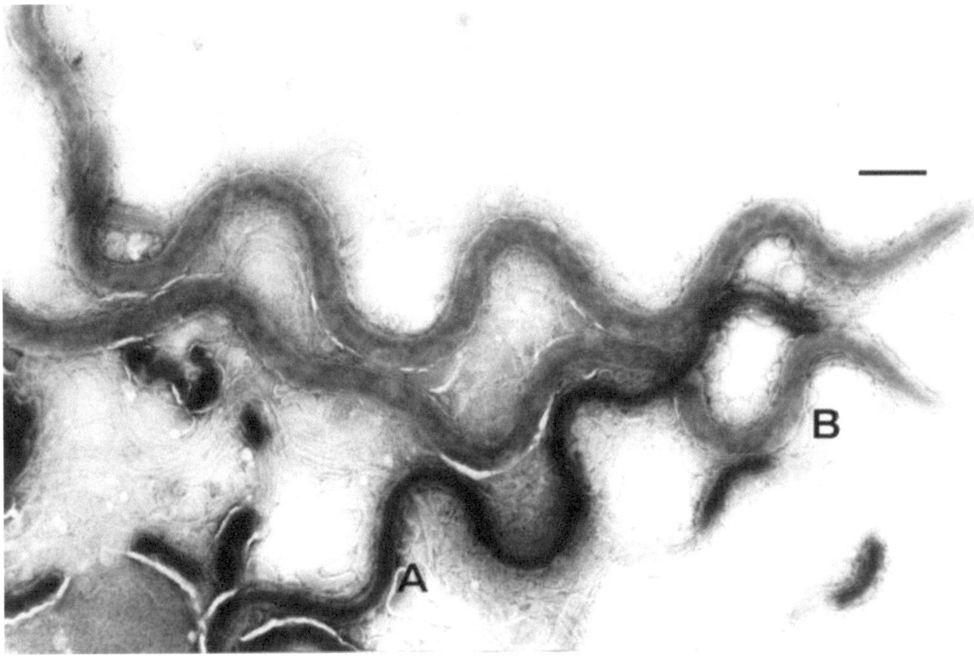

Fig. 5. Electron microscopy of unfixed, negative stained DK1 strain (skin isolate). This strain consist of two morphologically distinct borrelia A. small and B. larger *borrelia*. Bar 1 mm. Magnification 10,260 x.

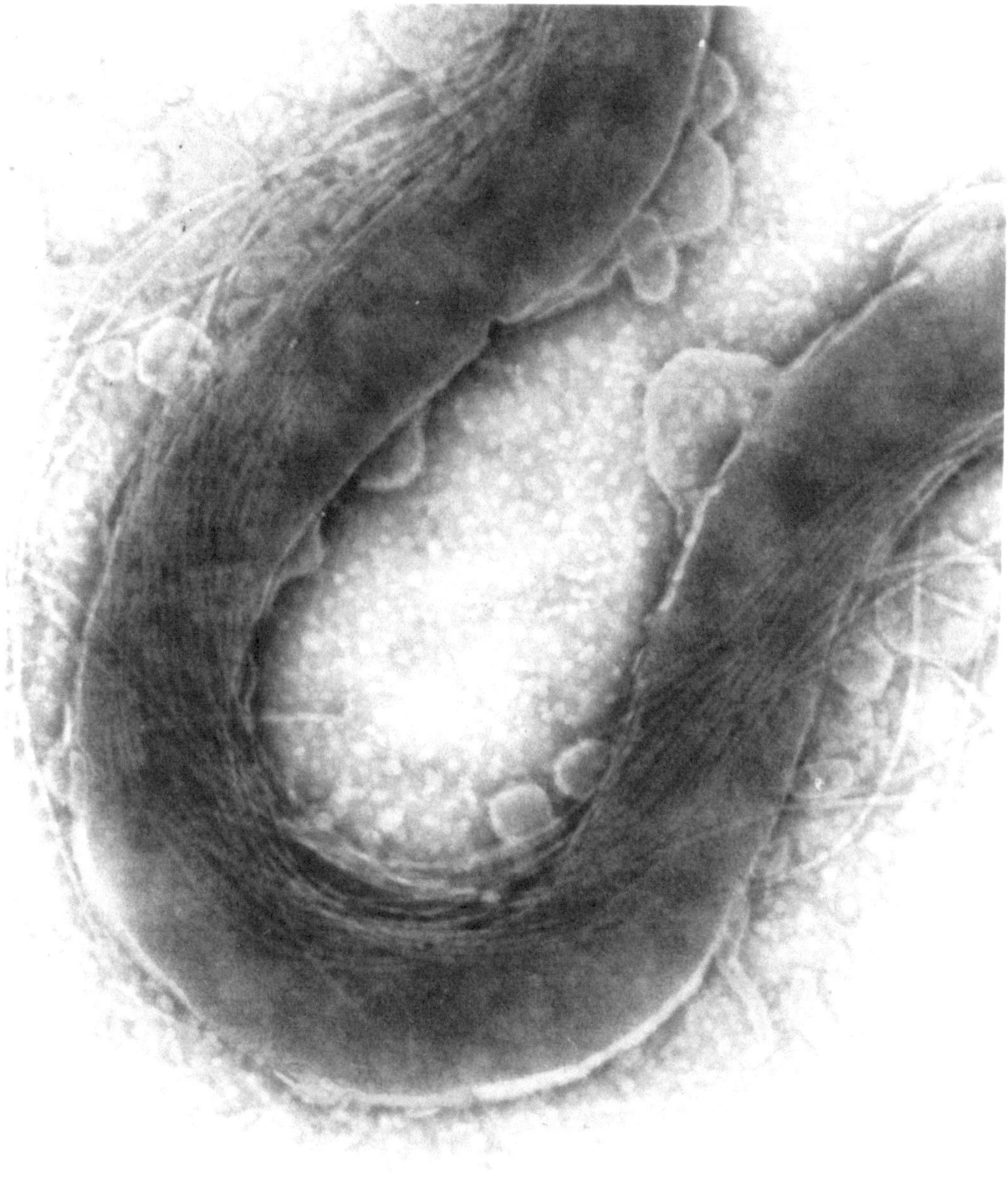

Fig. 6. Electron microscopy of unfixed, negative stained DK1 strain (skin isolate).

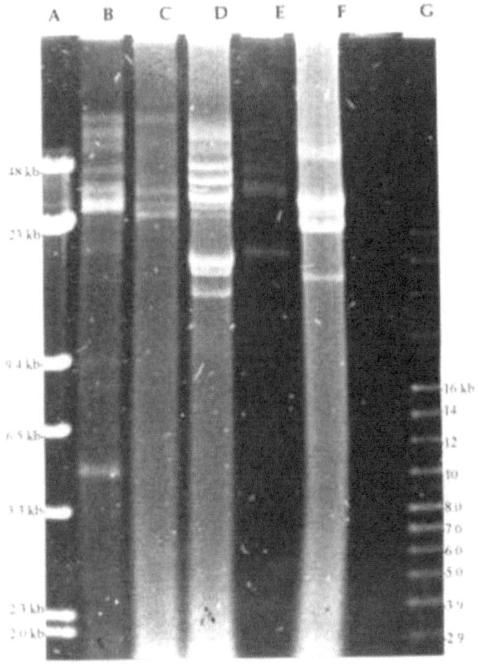

Fig. 7. Plasmids isolated from different strains of *Borrelia burgdorferi* : The Dk1 strain (B), Dk5 strain (C), DK6 strain (D), DK 2 strain (E), DK7 strain (F) and a super coiled circular molecular weight marker (G). Linear molecular markers (A) (HindIII fragments of Lambda DNA). Samples were separated in 0.3% gel at 14°C for 20 hr then stained with ethidium bromide.

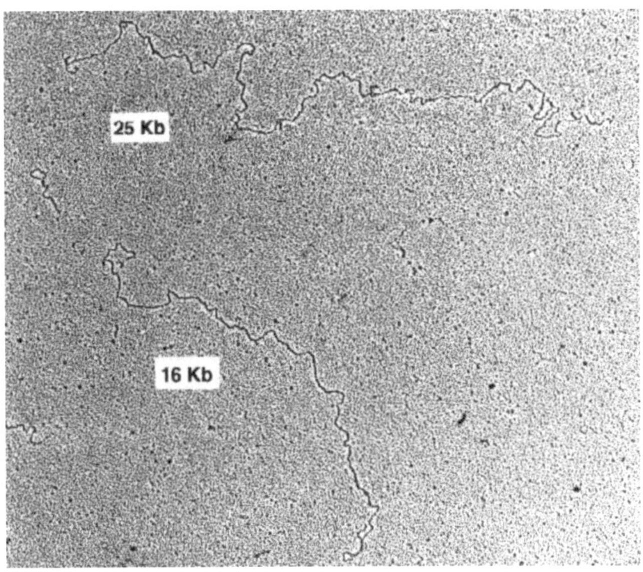

Fig. 8. Elrectron micrograph of 25 kb plasmid extracted from DK1 strain . One supercoiled plasmid. magnification 52000 x.

4. References

Burgdorfer W, Barbour AG, Hayes SF, Benach JL, Grunwaldt E, Davis JP (June 1982). "Lyme disease-a tick-borne spirochetosis?". Science 216 (4552): 1317–9.

Barbour, A.G. (1984) Isolation and cultivation of Lyme disease spirochetes. Yale J Biol Med 57: 521-525.

Barbour, A. G. & Garon, C. F., 1987. The Gene encoding major surface protein of *Borrelia burgdorferi* are located on a plasmid. Ann. NY. Acad. Sci., 539: 144-153.

Barbour, A. G. , 1988. *Plasmid analysis of Borrelia burgdorferi, the Lyme disease agent. : J. Clin.Microbiol., 26: 475-478.*

Barbour A.G. & Garon. C. F., 1987.Linear plasmids of the bacterium Borrelia burgdorferi have covalently closed ends. Science., 237: 409-411 .

Shigekawa, K., and Dower, W.J. (1988) Electroporation of eukaryotes and prokaryotes: a general approach to the introduction of macromolecules into cells. BioTechniques 6: 742-751.

Barbour, A. G., 1989.Classification of *Borrelia burgdorferi* on the basis of plasmid profiles. Zbl.Bakt.Supl.,18: 1-7.

Barbour. A. G., 1989.The Molecular biology of *Borrelia.* Rev .Infec.Disease. 11 suppl 6 s : 1470-1474.

Bergstrom. S. Bundoc. V. G & Barbour. A., 1989. Molecular analysis of linear plasmid - encoded major surface protein, OspA and OspB, of the lyme disease spirochaete *Borrelia burgdorferi*. Mol.microbiol.,3: 479-486.

Crespi, M., Messense, E. A Caplan, M. Von Montagu & Desomer, 1992. Fasciation Induction by the phytopatogen Rhodococoous fascians depends upon a linear plasmid Encoding a cytokinin synthase gene. EMBO. J., 11: 795-804.

Davidson .B. E, Mac Dugall J & Girons. I. S., 1992. Physical map of the linear chromosome of the bacterium *Borrelia burgdorferi*, a causative agent of lyme disease, and localization of rRNA Genes. J.Bacteriol., 174: 3766-3774.

Ferdows .M. S, Barbour .A. G., 1989.Megabase-sized linear DNA in the bacterium Borrelia burgdorferi, the lyme disease agent. Proc.Natl. Acad.Sci.USA., 86: 5969-5973.

Hansen, K., hovmark, A., Lebech,A .m., Lebech,k., Olsson,I., Halkier,l ;et al. 1992. Roxithromycin in Lyme borreliosis: discrepant Results of in vitro and in vivo animal susceptibility study and clinical trial in patients with erythema migrans. Acta.Derm.Venerol., 72: 297-300.

Hinnebusch. J & Barbour. A. G., 1991.Linear plasmids of Borrelia burgdorferi have a telomeric structure and sequence similar to those of eukaryotic virus. J. Bacteriol., 173: 7233-7239.

Schwan.T. G, Burgdorfer. W. & Garon. C. F ., 1988. Change in Infectivity and Plasmid Profile of Lyme Disease Spirochete, Borrelia Borgdorferi, as a Result of In vitro cultivation. Inf. Immun ., 56: 1831-1836.

Servent, A. A., Charachon, S, Y., Bilak,E, J., Karayan, L. & Ramuz .M., 1993. Presence of one linear and one circular chromosome in the Agrobacterium tumefaciens C58 genome. J. bacteriol., 175: 7869-7874.

Sherwood, C & Wai .M.H.,1993. Linear chromosomal and genetic map of Borrelia burgdorferi, the lyme disease Agent. Molecular miccrobiol., 8 (5): 967-980.

A G Barbour, C J Carter, V Bundoc, and J Hinnebusch. The nucleotide sequence of a linear plasmid of Borrelia burgdorferi reveals similarities to those of circular plasmids of other prokaryotes.J Bacteriol. 1996 November; 178(22): 6635–6639.

Fraser CM, Casjens S, Huang WM, et al. (December 1997). "Genomic sequence of a Lyme disease spirochaete, Borrelia burgdorferi". Nature 390 (6660): 580–6.

Bundoc, V.G., and Barbour, A.G. (1989) Clonal polymorphisms of outer membrane protein OspB of *Borrelia burgdorferi*. Infect Immun 57: 2733-2741.

Hinnebusch, J., and Tilly, K. (1993) Linear plasmids and chromosomes in bacteria. Mol Microbiol 10: 917-922.

Rosa, P., Samuels, D.S., Hogan, D., Stevenson, B., Casjens, S., and Tilly, K. (1996) Directed insertion of a selectable marker into acircular plasmid of *Borrelia burgdorferi*. J Bacteriol 178: 5946-5953.

Saint Girons, I., Old, I.G., and Davidson, B.E. (1994) Molecular biology of the Borrelia, bacteria with linear replicons. Microbiology 140: 1803-1816.

Samuels, D.S., and Garon, C.F. (1993) Coumermycin A1 inhibits growth and induces relaxation of supercoiled plasmids in *Borrelia burgdorferi*, the Lyme disease agent. Antimicrob Agents Chemother 37: 46-50.

Tilly, K., Casjens, S., Stevenson, B., Bono, J., Samuels, D.S., Hogan, D. and Rosa, P. (1997) The *Borrelia burgdorferi* circular plasmid cp26: conservation of plasmid structure and targeted inactivation of the *ospC* gene. Mol. Microbiol. 25:361-373.

Ali Karami , Peter Hindeersson , Niels Hoiby , Saeid Morovvati and Akbar Khalilpour. Linear and Circular Plasmids in Skin and Cerebrospinal Fluid Isolates of Borrelia burgdorferi Agent of Lyme Disease. Pakistan Journal of Biological Sciences 2006 (9): 15 ,2787-2793

Ali KARAMI, Seyed Mohammad Javad HOSSEYNI, Yaser KIARUDI .Molecular Characterization of Borrelia burgdorferi Linear Plasmids by DNA Hybridization, PCR, Two-Dimensional Gel Electrophoresis, and Electron Microscopy. Turk J Biol 31 (2007) 73-80.

A Karami, P Hindersson, N Høiby, S Morovvati. OspA Sequence Comparison and Protection Against Borrelia burgdorferi Infection in Gerbils by Recombinant OspA Protein. Iranian Journal of Public Health 2006;35(2):16-24.

Sorouri R, Ranjbar R, Jonaidi Jafari N, Karami A. Rapid detection of Borrelia burgdorferi strains by nested polymerase chain reaction. Pak J Biol Sci. 2009 Mar 1;12(5):463-6.

Galdwin, Mark; Trattler, Bill (2009). Spirochetes: Clinical Microbiology Made Ridiculously Simple. MedMaster, Inc. ISBN 978-0-940780-81-1.

Samuels DS; Radolf, JD. (2010). Borrelia: Molecular Biology, Host Interaction and Pathogenesis. Caister Academic Press. ISBN 978-1-904455-58-5.

2

Zoonotic Peculiarities of *Borrelia burgdorferi* s.l.: Vectors Competence and Vertebrate Host Specificity

Alexandru Movila[1], Ion Toderas[1], Helen V. Dubinina[2], Inga Uspenskaia[1] and Andrey N. Alekseev[2]
[1]*Institute of Zoology, Moldova Academy of Science*
[2]*Zoological Institute, Russia Academy of Science*
[1]*Republic of Moldova*
[2]*Russia Federation*

1. Introduction

Tick-borne diseases are of increasing public health concern because of range expansions of both vectors and pathogens (Daniel et al., 2003). Lyme borreliosis is the most common arthropod-borne human disease in temperate regions of the northern hemisphere. The causative agents of Lyme borreliosis (and other tick-borne borrelioses) are spirochaetes belonging to the *Borrelia burgdorferi* sensu lato (s.l.) species complex. It is well known that *B. burgdorferi* are unique among the pathogenic spirochaetes by requiring obligate blood-feeding arthropods for their transmission and maintenance in vertebrate host populations. All known causative agents of borrelioses circulate between ticks (Arachnida, Acari, Ixodoidea) and wide variety of vertebrates species (mammals, birds and reptiles). Consequently, *Borrelia* populations are shaped by the dynamics and demographic processes of host and vector populations, host and vector immune responses and extrinsic abiotic factors (e.g. combination of temperature, humidity and types of climate and landscape) affecting host and vector populations (Margos et al., 2011).

The main goals of this chapter are to summarize the results of vector competence analyses and vertebrate hosts' specificity for Lyme disease agents, give a general description of *B. burgdorferi* (s.l.)—tick—vertebrate hosts relationships in natural foci.

2. *Borrelia burgdorferi* s.l. genospecies diversity and association with vectors and reservoirs

From the time of *B. burgdorferi* discovery a large number of *Borrelia* isolates has been obtained from various vertebrate species, including humans. Involvements of other species from the *B. burgdorferi* s.l. complex were recognized recently. *Borrelia* spirochaetes are transmitted to reservoirs (including humans) by all 3 developmental stages of ixodid ticks (Fig 1 A), but the nymphal stage appears to be the most important at least in the North America and West Europe (Anderson et al., 1990; Kurtenbach et al., 1998; Kurtenbach et al., 2006).Considering

Borrelia species	Vector	Reservoirs	Geographical distribution	Reference
1-st group				
B. afzelii	*Ixodes ricinus, Ixodes persulcatus*	Rodents	Asia, Europe	Canica et al. (1993)
B. bavariensis	*Ixodes ricinus*	Rodents	Europe	Margos et al. (2009)
B. bissettii	*Ixodes ricinus, Ixodes scapularis, Ixodes pacificus, Ixodes minor*	Rodents	Europe, United States	Postic et al. (1998)
B. burgdorferi sensu stricto	*Ixodes ricinus, Ixodes scapularis, Ixodes pacificus, Ixodes persulcatus*	Rodents, birds, lizards, big mammals	Europe, United States, Asia	Baranton et al. (1992); Alekseev et al. (2010)
B. garinii	*Ixodes ricinus, Ixodes persulcatus, Ixodes hexagonus, Ixodes nipponensis, Ixodes pavlovskyi, Ixodes trianguliceps*	Birds, lizards, rodents	Asia, Europe	Baranton et al. (1992); Gorelova et al. (1996); Korenberg et al. (2010)
B. kurtenbachii	*Ixodes scapularis*	Rodents	Europe, United States	Margos et al. (2010)
B. lusitaniae	*Ixodes ricinus, Ixodes persulcatus*	Rodents, lizards	Europe, North Africa	Le Fleche et al. (1997); Alekseev et al. (2010)
B. spielmanii	*Ixodes ricinus*	Rodents	Europe	Richter et al. (2004, 2006)
B. valaisiana	*Ixodes ricinus, Ixodes granulatus, Ixodes persulcatus*	Birds, lizards	Asia, Europe	Wang et al. (1997); Alekseev et al. (1998, 2010)
2-nd group				
B. americana	*Ixodes pacificus, Ixodes minor*	Birds	United States	Rudenko et al. (2009b)
B. andersonii	*Ixodes dentatus*	Cotton tail rabbit	United States	Marconi et al. (1995)
B. californiensis	*Ixodes pacificus, Ixodes jellisoni, Ixodes spinipalpis*	Kangaroo rat, mule deer	United States	Postic et al. (2007)

Borrelia species	Vector	Reservoirs	Geographical distribution	Reference
B. carolinensis	*Ixodes minor*	Rodents, birds	United States	Rudenko et al. (2009a)
B. japonica	*Ixodes ovatus*	Rodents	Japan	Kawabata et al. (1993)
B. sinica	*Ixodes ovatus*	Rodents	China	Masuzawa et al. (2001)
B. tanukii	*Ixodes tanuki*	Unknown (possibly dogs and cats)	Japan	Fukunaga et al. (1996)
B. turdi	*Ixodes turdus*	Birds	Japan	Fukunaga et al. (1996b)
B. yangtze	*Ixodes granulatus, Haemaphysalis longicornis*	Rodents	China	Chu et al. (2008)
3-rd group				
Genomospecies 2	*Ixodes pacificus*	Unknown	United States	Postic et al. (2007)

Table 1. Currently known species from the Borrelia burgdorferi sensu lato complex (Rudenko et al., 2011 with modifications)

the human sensitivity to *B. burgdorferi* s.l. and results of the newest publications, the complex of 18 *Borrelia* species (Table 1) can be divided into 3 major groups (Rudenko et al., 2011): the first and second groups contains 9 species with pathogenic potential and species that have not yet been reported in or isolated from humans, respectively, and the 3rd still not named group proposed as genomospecies 2 represented by two far-western US isolates.

3. Ticks–Borreliae interface

3.1 Vectors ecological groups

There are two big ecological groups of tick species. Ticks seek hosts by an interesting behaviour called "questing." Questing ticks (=exophilic, polyxenous) crawl up the stems of grass or perch on the edges of leaves on the ground in a typical posture with the front legs extended, especially in response to a host passing by (Fig. 1 A). In contrast to questing ticks, nidicolous (=endophilic, mainly monoxenous) ticks live in secluded enclosures such as caves, burrows and nests of their hosts or harborages near these nests (Fig. 1 B, C) (Sonenshine, 1991).

3.2 Vector competence for *Borrelia burgdorferi* s.l.

The primary vectors of Lyme borreliosis spirochaetes to humans in temperate regions of the northern hemisphere are closely taxonomically related tick species: *I. pacificus* in Western North America, *I. persulcatus* in Eurasia, *I. ricinus* in Europe and *I. scapularis* in eastern North

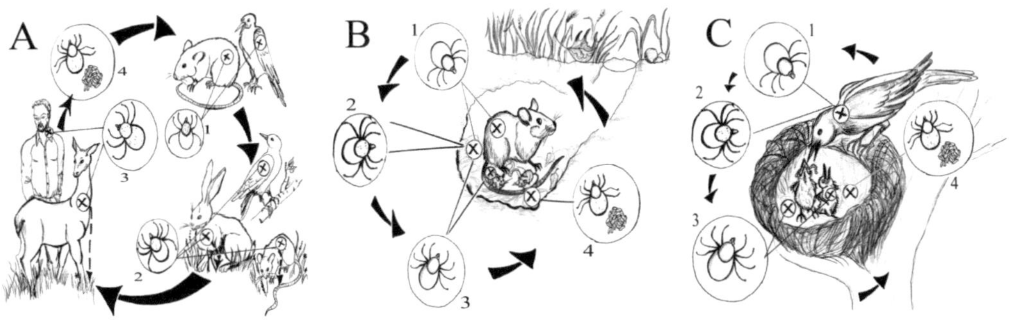

Fig. 1. The life circles of exophilic and endophilic ticks. A - exophilic tick life cycle, B - mammals-associated endophilic life cycle; C - bird-associated endophilic life cycle. 1 - Larvae, 2 - Nymph, 3 - Adult, 4 - Female with eggs

America. These ticks are basically forest dwellers, spending most of their time hiding in the leaf litter of the forest floor, where humidity is high and the risk of dehumidification is low. Ticks require three hosts, and their life cycle takes between 1-3 years to complete. The immature stages (larvae and nymphs) of the tick quest on low lying vegetation and tend to infest smaller hosts to obtain their blood meals, especially rodents, insectivores and birds. After feeding, they detach from their host and molt to the next development stage (larvae to nymph or nymph to adult tick) on the ground under leafs and other kind of the litter. The adult ticks have sexual dimorphism and only females take a big amount of blood meal, whereas males [at least *I. persulcatus* (Alekseev, 1992)] take a small amount of blood but nevertheless can transmit TBEV to human (for review see Alekseev et al., 2010). Both sexes tend to quest up on vegetations and generally infest different species of ungulates, carnivores and lagomorphs. After feeding, the female lay one batch of thousands of eggs and then die. Only one blood meal is taken during each of the three life stages.

In many ways, these ticks are ideally suited as vectors of zoonotic pathogens, since they feed on wide variety of animals but also include humans within the range of hosts they willing feed upon (Filippova, 1977; Xu et al., 2003).

To date, vector competence for *B. burgdorferi* s.l. has been experimentally confirmed for 12 tick species: *Ixodes affinis* Neumann, *Ixodes jellisoni* Cooley & Kohls, *Ixodes pacificus* Cooley & Kohls, *Ixodes persulcatus* Schulze, *Ixodes ricinus* (Linnaeus), *Ixodes scapularis* Say, *Ixodes angustus* Neumann, *Ixodes dentatus* Marx, *Ixodes hexagonus* Leach, *Ixodes minor* Neumann, *Ixodes muris* Bishopp & Smith and *Ixodes spinipalpis* Hadwen & Nuttall. Published vector competence studies have included only four *B. burgdorferi* s.l. genospecies (*B. burgdorferi* s.s., *B. afzelii*, *B. bissettii*, *B. garinii*) (Eisen & Lane, 2002).

The majority of the remaining confirmed vectors feed primary on rodents and/or lagomorphs (i.e. *I. dentatus*, *I. jellisoni*, *I. muris* and *I. spinipalpis* in North America and *I. minor* in North and South America), whereas *I. affinis* infests a wide variety of mammals in North and South America; *I. hexagonus* being a nidicolous arthropod is found on various medium sized mammals in Europe and north-western Africa (Jaenson et al., 1994). Their host preferences and ***modus vivendi*** render these tick species unlikely to act as vectors to humans.

In addition to the experimentally confirmed vectors, the presence of *Borrelia* in ticks and their primary hosts suggest vector competence for *B. burgdorferi* s.l. of several other *Ixodes* spp. These includes the avian-associated nidicolous tick species such as *Ixodes uriae* White (Olsen et al., 1995), *Ixodes lividus* Koch (Movila et al., 2008), *Ixodes arboricola* Schulze & Schlottke (Špitalská et al., 2011), *Ixodes auritulus* Neumann (Morshed et al., 2005), *Ixodes turdus* Nakatsuji (Fukunaga et al., 1996a) and mammals-associated nidicolous ticks - *Ixodes trianguliceps* Birula (Gorelova et al., 1996) and *Ixodes neotomae* Cooley (Schwan et al., 1993).

Seven tick species evaluated for vector competence appear unable to transmit *B. burgdorferi* s.l.: *Amblyomma americanum* (Linnaeus), *Dermacentor andersoni* Stiles, *Dermacentor occidentalis* Marx, *Dermacentor variabilis* (Say), *Ixodes cookie* Packard, *Ixodes holocyclus* Neumann and *Ixodes ovatus* Neumann. In most cases these ticks acquired borreliae better feeding on infected hosts but transstadial passage was rare or absent, and there was no evidence of spirochaetes transmission during feeding (Eisen & Lane, 2002).

Taken all data together, there are 3 kinds of *Borrelia* species and vectors competence:

1. Those associated with a vector characterized by both a broad spectrum of hosts *(I. ricinus, I. persulcatus* or *I. scapularis)* and by a huge expansion area. These species have large populations of individuals and a variety of different vertebrate hosts which do not fully characterize the concerned *Borrelia* species. These species are genetically quite diverse and usually pathogenic or potentially pathogenic (*B. burgdorferi* s.s., *B. garinii, B. afzelii, B. valaisiana, B. lusitaniae,* etc.).
2. A second kind of species associated with either a unique reservoir or a unique specialized vector *(B. andersonii, B. turdi, B. tanukii)*, or an unspecialized vector but still a unique reservoir (*B. spielmanii)*.
3. Incompetence vector species. Mátlová et al. (1996) showed that unlike *I. ricinus, Dermacentor reticulatus* (Fabricius) reveals a gradual decline and the loss of Lyme borrelioses spirochaetes shortly after infection. This indicates a lack of this ixodid species to serve as a competent vector of *B. burgdorferi*.

Thus, the physiological mechanisms of vector competence in various tick species remain to be explained and require further studies.

3.3 Ticks behaviour and *Borrelia* transmission

Ticks can survive for years in their biotopes; however, they spend only a small part of their life in a parasitic phase. Most of the *Ixodes* spp. lifetime is spent outside of the hosts, either on the vegetation, ground or in the litter.

To find a host, *I. ricinus* climbs onto low vegetation and waits at the tip where they quest for a host for time-limited periods. During these periods of questing, ticks stay mainly immobile at the tip of the vegetation. When ticks are questing, they respond to mechanical and chemical stimuli produced by hosts, including humans. When hosts pass close enough, questing ticks grab their hosts but sometimes crawl in the direction of the possible prey. Such behaviour of *I. ricinus* is important since it implies that hosts, including humans, take some active part in the tick-host encounter. So, the successful transmission of pathogens to humans depends on the behaviour of the vectors.

Methods used to estimate tick behaviour vary and are generally directed to ascertain locomotor activity, which implies an orientation to physical parameters of the environment such as relative humidity, temperature, light and behaviour during questing for a host.

The predominant behaviour of *I. ricinus* is the tendency of the tick to ascend vegetation during the day and descent at night (Lees & Milne, 1951), while Okulova (1978) showed that *I. persulcatus* adults climbed up the aconite and fern stems to a maximum height of 80 cm (according to observations of Filippova (1977) some of *I. persulcatus* specimens in Primorye (Russian Far East) climb to a height of 2 m) when the temperature is 23.3° C. The maximum activity of *I. ricinus* larvae and adults was associated with the lightest part of the day, 1 p.m., when the air temperature was highest; the adults increased activity of females was observed between 1 p.m and 8 p.m. (Dubinina & Makrushina, 1997). Babenko (1985) suggested the crepuscular activity of ticks to be adaptive, coinciding with the activity of hosts they feed on.

Alekseev et al. (1998) reported that different *Borrelia* genospecies prevailed during different periods of the tick activity season. The author showed that *Borrelia*-infected nymphs and adults emerged within a day later than uninfected ticks and only after 11 a.m., when the temperature gradient exceeded 0.5° C. On the basis of these data Prof. Alekseev proposed a hypothesis that the response of *Borrelia*-infected *I. persulcatus* ticks to some external factors (plant and animal odors) was different from that of the uninfected ticks.

Lefcort & Durden (1996) studied the behaviour of *I. scapularis* nymphs and adults, and compared specimens that were infected in the laboratory by *B. burgdorferi* s.s. to uninfected ticks. The authors showed a stimulating effect of Borreliae on the activity of tick nymphs.

However the work of Alekseev et al. (2000) may be the most interesting example of the behaviour of infected and naive *I. persulcatus* and *I. ricinus* ticks. The comparison of *I. persulcatus* and *I. ricinus* demonstrated that the entire locomotor activity of *I. persulcatus* nymphs was 4 times and that of adults approximately 2 times as great as that of *I. ricinus*. The activity of infected preimaginal and adults *I. ricinus* was less than that of uninfected ticks. These report support earliest opinion that the *I. persulcatus* ticks are more effective vectors of pathogens than *I. ricinus* (Alekseev & Dubinina, 1994; Kovalevskii & Korenberg, 1995). Interesting, the European *Borrelia* genospecies depressed the nymphal activity of *I. ricinus* and *I. persulcatus* ticks. The data of Alekseev et al. (2000) and Lefcort & Durden (1996) can explain the role of nymphs as major vector of Lyme disease in North America and adults - in Euro-Asia.

The group of prof. Alekseev A.N. (for review see Alekseev et al., 2010) demonstrated that adults having exoskeleton anomalies (Fig. 2) and *Borrelia* infection moved more actively than ticks with normal morphology and with infection. This anomalies ticks phenomenon appeared to be associated with the consequences of the anthropogenic pressure and with environmental pollution, which caused the development of tick population with changed morphology and metabolism. It is clear that the accumulation of these anomalies ticks in the vector population increased the risk of pathogen transmission.

The ability of anomalous and normal ticks to attack humans was tested by Alekseev & Dubinina (2006). During 25 minutes of the experiments, none of the normal females attached onto the human skin, while anomalous females started as earlier as 1 minute after the release and this process was painless. The attachment sites of the ticks were corresponded to the acupuncture points on the human body with the impedance 172 ± 3.2 kΩ (Alekseev & Dubinina, 2006). The fact that ticks attach to different sites on the body of the same person perhaps reflects the temporal changes in impedance (Alekseev et al., 2010). The ticks with anomalous in exoskeleton contain heavy metals in their bodies (especially Cd) are more sensitive in their impedance measurements. The attachment of the anomalous female may be an indicator of a higher aggressiveness exhibited by anomalous, even pathogen-free ticks to humans.

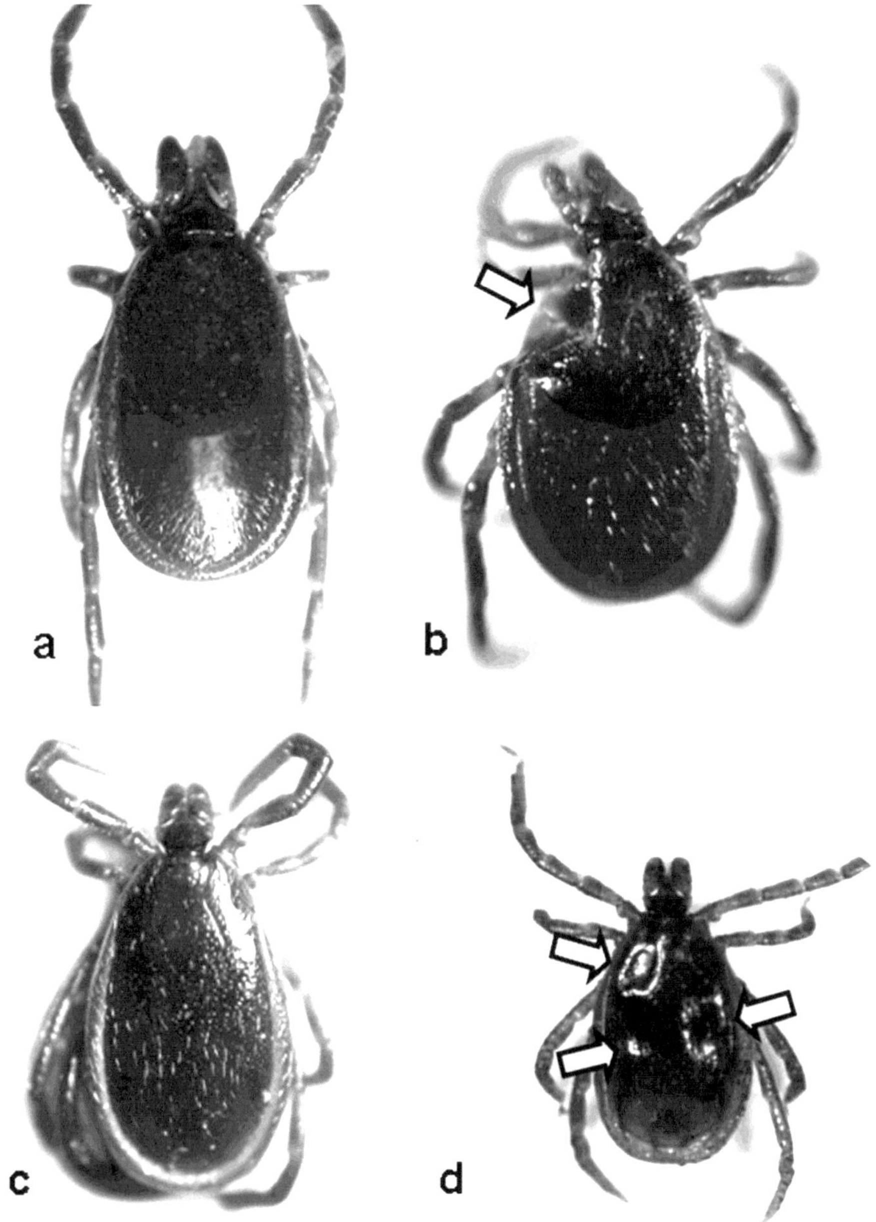

Fig. 2. Adult *Ixodes persulcatus* ticks, collected in vicinities of St. Petersburg (North-West Russia). Females: normal (a), anomalous (b); males: normal (c), anomalous (d). Arrows indicate prominent cuticular depressions symptomatic of exoskeleton pathologies in anomalous ticks (Original photos)

When unfed *I. ricinus* attaches to a vertebrate host, *Borrelia* transmission does not occur at the beginning of the blood uptake but later on, and transmission efficiency increases with the duration of the blood meal (Crippa et al., 2002; Kahl et al., 1998). The delay in transmission observed during the first hours of the blood meal might be due to this phenomenon, the migration of the spirochaetes from midgut to salivary glands. Crippa et al. (2002), comparing transmission dynamic of spirochaetes by *B. burgdorferi* s.s.- and *B. afzelii*-infected ticks, reported that this delay might also be influenced by the *Borrelia* species infecting the ticks. In fact, earlier transmission occurred when ticks were infected by *B. afzelii* rather than by *B. burgdorferi* s.s. These authors reported that during the first 48 h of attachment to the host, *B. burgdorferi* s.s.-infected ticks did not infect the 18 exposed mice, whereas *B. afzelii*-infected ticks transmitted infection to 33% of the mice. This study not only showed that *I. ricinus* transmits *B. afzelii* earlier than *B. burgdorferi* s.s., but also that *I. ricinus* is a more efficient vector for *B. afzelii* than for *B. burgdorferi* s.s. Unfortunately, nothing is known on the transmission delay for other pathogenic *Borrelia* species infecting *I. ricinus*, such as *B. garinii*, *B. valaisiana* and the recently described species *B. spielmanii*.

Whereas *B. burgdorferi* transmission to the host usually does not occur during the first 40 h of the blood meal in the North American vector ticks *I. scapularis* and *I. pacificus* (Peavey & Lane, 1995; Piesman et al., 1987, 1991), while *I. ricinus* nymphs were shown to be capable of transmitting *B. burgdorferi* s.l. to mongolian gerbils as early as within the first 24 h of feeding (Kahl et al., 1998). There is a method that allows assessment of the duration of tick feeding as a basis for determining the individual risk of *B. burgdorferi* transmission to the person bitten by a tick. Piesman & Spielman (1980) were the first to establish the so-called scutal index as a quick and simple measure of engorgement and feeding time in partially fed *I. scapularis* nymphs. The scutal index is the ratio between length of the tick alloscutum (a) and width of scutum (b) (Fig. 3).Falco et al. (1996) reported that the scutual index of *I. scapularis* nymphs detached from humans was on average equality to 34.7 h post-attachment. Yeh et al. (1995) reported that only 10% and 41% of people had found and removed *I. scapularis* nymphs by 24 h and 36 h of attachment, respectively. The situation is probably similar in Europe, but there is one important difference: whereas North American tick bite victims have a very good chance to avoid *Borrelia* infection after a tick bite lasting approximately 36 h, many *I. ricinus* nymphs might already have transmitted borreliae to their host after this feeding time.

Meiners et al. (2006) reported that a scutal index of 1.1 as a cutoff allows a clear distinction between high-risk versus low-risk group ticks. The large majority of *I. ricinus* nymphs with a scutal index <1.1 may have fed for <24 h, and the resulting risk of *B. burgdorferi* transmission and host infection might be low, even in the case of a *B. burgdorferi*-infected tick. The risk of host infection might be distinctly higher when a *B. burgdorferi*-infected *I. ricinus* nymph has a scutal index 1.1–1.5 (corresponding to ~24 – ~40 h feeding duration). Infection risk might be very high, if the detached tick has a scutal index >1.5 indicating that it might have fed for >36 h. Sood et al. (1997) identified a long feeding duration in *I. scapularis* ticks as a major risk indicator of *B. burgdorferi* host infection. Influence of borreliae on the salivary gland genome results the appearance of proteins, which suppress vertebrate immune system and properties of *Borrelia*.

Among vast family of proteins derived from tick salivary glands as a result of its genome activity the most interesting multifunctional one is presented by so called salp15 (14.7 kDa).

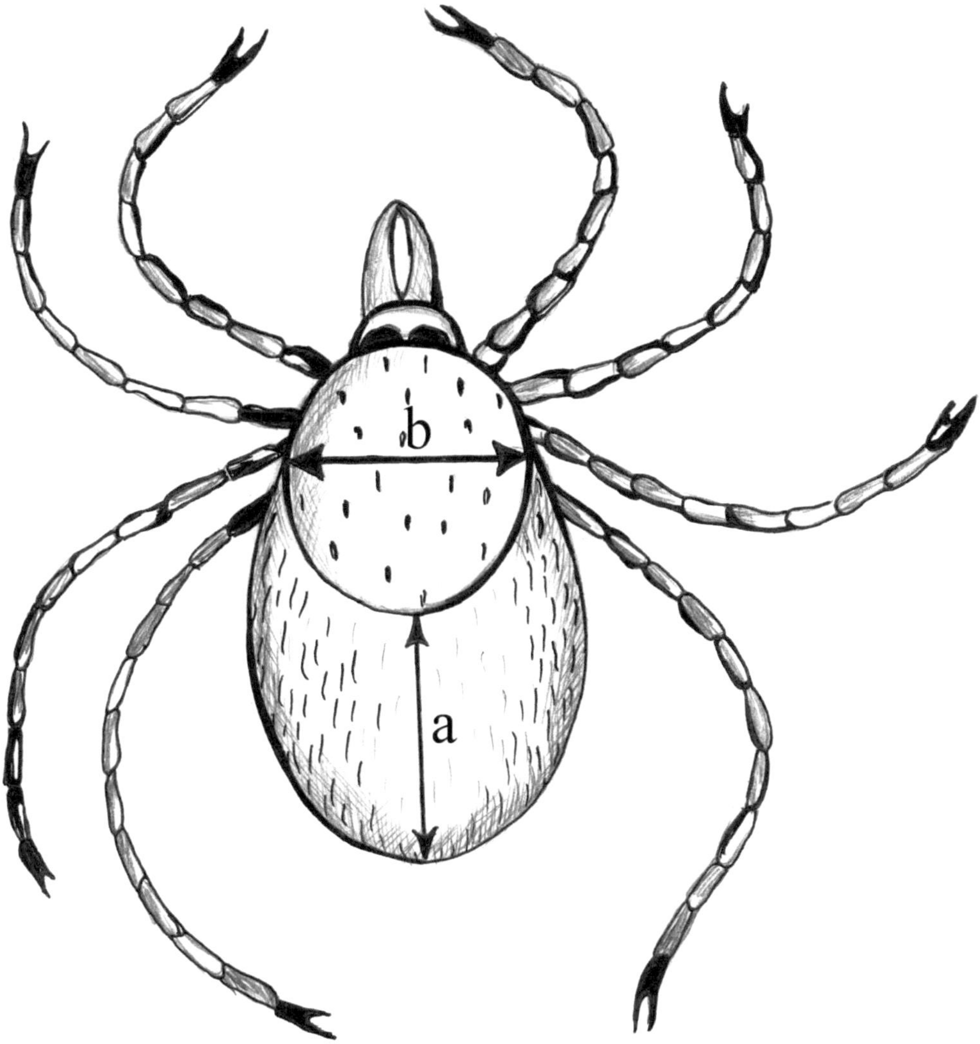

Fig. 3. Scutual index (= a/b) of *Ixodes ricinus* nymphs (Meiners et al., 2006)

Actions of this protein have two directions: the first one channeled on vertebrate immune system suppression, the second one directed on infection enlighten of both pathogenic for human microorganism hosts. The first one is working independently of the presents of pathogenic for human microorganisms. The second one is working in dependence of infection. For example *I. scapularis* salp15 inhibits CD4+ T-cell activation (Anguita et al., 2002) by binding to the CD4 receptor (Garg et al., 2006). Hovius and his colleagues (Hovius et al., 2008) found that salp15 from the same species of tick is able to bind the C-type lectin DC-SIGN on human dendritic cells. Such binding inhibits cytokine expression by impairing both nucleosome remodeling and mRNA stabilizations. All these mechanisms are functioning without borreliae action.

It is known now that the presence of OspC facilitates *B. burgdorferi* invasion of *I. scapularis* salivary glands. Pal et al. (2004), Rudenko et al. (2005) affirmed that in the beginning of infected (OspA) vertebrate' blood consuming borreliae enhanced salp15 production, which lighten tick infection. Just the opposite action, in which salp15 is also included, consist in prevention of *B. burgdorferi* infected (OspC) tick saliva from killing by anti-OspC antibodies in the tick just after beginning of attachment and feeding (Ramamoorthi et al., 2005). Rosa (2005) naming his article "Lyme disease agent borrows a practical coat" meaning that coat helped spirochaetes "to change into a new suit" and transfer themselves into the vertebrate host.

In the interface of field collected *I. ricinus* infected by different quantity of representatives of 4 species *Borrelia* determined by real time PCR and RLB a very interesting fact was discovered: the better surviving of adult ticks infected by mean doses of pathogens (Herrmann & Gern, 2010). This phenomenon was a brilliant confirmation of prof. Alekseev (1984) theory that among other criteria of interface specificity in the couple "vector—pathogen" the existence of optimum pathogen doses (mean ones) do exist not only in the pairs *"Leishmania – sand flies"*, plague agent and fleas (Alekseev, 1984), "Tick-borne encephalitis (TBE) virus —*Ixodes persulcatus*" (Alekseev & Kondrashova, 1985), but in the couple *"Borrelia – Ixodes ticks"* (Herrmann & Gern, 2010).

3.4 *Borrelia* circulation in tick population

Ticks may acquire various *Borrelia* species through their successive blood meals on various hosts, and maintain the infection to the subsequent stage via transstadial transmission: larvae—nymph—adult.

Transovarial transmission of infection agents, which is an important factor of maintaining the disease foci, depends not only on the female obtaining the infection agents at the previous developmental stage, but also on the female contacting the infected male. The success of these contacts, and thus the probability of transmission, is based on the details of the sexual behaviour of the vectors. According to available data, which are scarce and often insufficiently representative, the frequency of *Borrelia* transovarial transmission in Lyme disease main vectors (*I. ricinus, I. persulcatus* and *I. scapularis*) may vary but never was estimated as frequent phenomenon (Du et al., 1990; Dubinina, 2000; Lane & Burgdorfer, 1987; Nakao & Miyamoto, 1992; Nefedova et al., 2004). On the basis of published data, probably, this transmission pathway apparently plays no significant role in the maintenance of *Borrelia* circulation and the dynamics of parameters of infection in adult ticks of the next generation. Nevertheless, transovarially transmitted spirochaetes may also contribute to mixed infections in ticks (Gern, 2009). However, *Borrelia miyamotoi* (a relapsing fever spirochete) is transmitted transovarially in *Ixodes* ticks and occurs sympatrically with *B. burgdorferi* spirochaetes (Piesman, 2002).

Thus, mixed infection with more than one species in ticks can be observed in some European endemic areas. These multiple infections may result from the tick species feeding on a host infected by more than one *Borrelia* species or from infected ticks feeding simultaneously with uninfected ticks on a host and exchanging the *Borrelia* species through co-feeding transmission from infected to uninfected ticks (Fig. 4). Different combinations of mixed infections with 2 or 3 species have been detected in *I. ricinus*. *Borrelia garinii* and

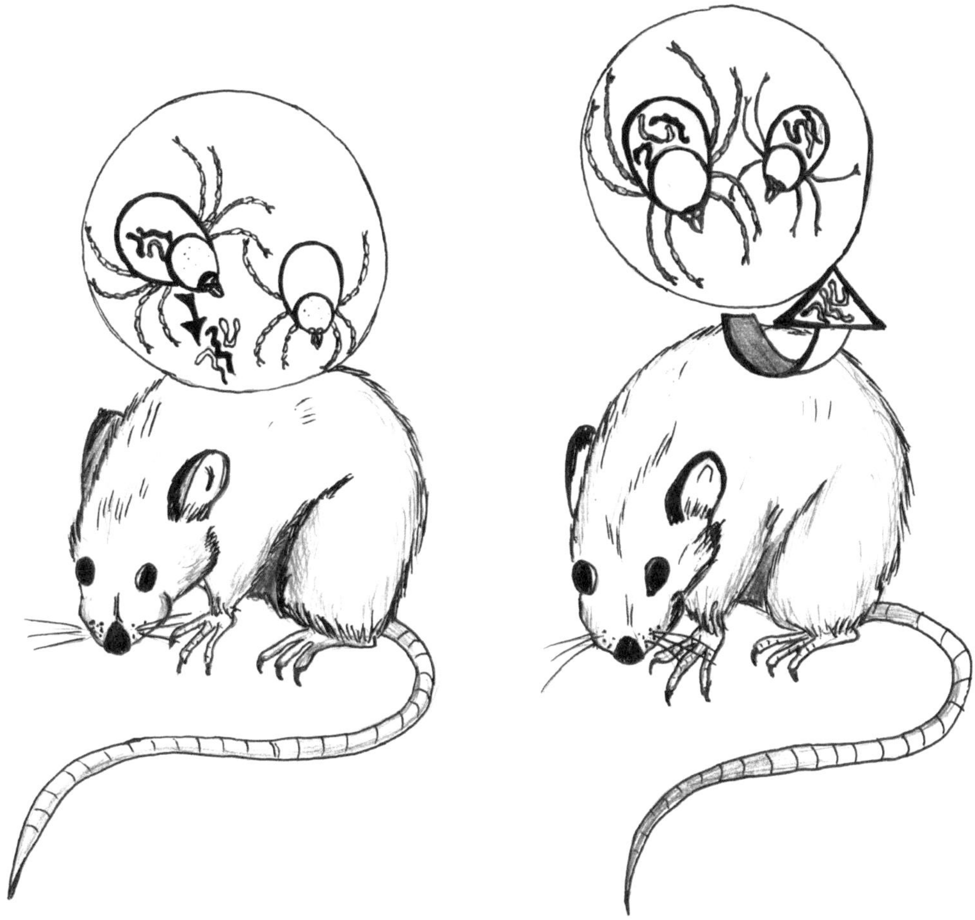

Fig. 4. *Borrelia* spp. co-feeding transmission

B. valaisiana constitute the majority of mixed infections, followed by mixed infections with *B. garinii* and *B. afzelii.* Such mixed infections are reported less frequently than single infections, and are often detected by PCR.

Ticks also can get *Borrelia* during copulation. Sexual transmission of microbial pathogens is a well-known phenomenon in arthropods. It was first described in soft ticks (Ornithodorinae) for relapsing fever *Borrelia* (Gaber et al., 1982, 1984; Wagner-Jevseenko, 1958). Chunikhin et al. (1983) studied the sexual transmission of the (TBE) virus in *I. persulcatus*. The virus was transmitted from the infected male tick to the female tick and was present in spermatocytes and spermatids of male ticks (Stefutkina, 1989). TBE virus was subsequently detected in the ovaries of 10% of the infected female ticks. Alekseev et al. (1999) have demonstrated that *B. garinii (*but not *B. afzelii)* spirochaetes can be transmitted from male to female in *I. persulcatus* ticks during copulation. Transmission of *B. garinii* to the female tick was observed more often when the male tick carried high numbers of spirochaetes. This observation is in accordance with the fact that ticks which carry high numbers of spirochaetes in the gut show systemic infection (i.e. outside the gut lumen) more often than ticks which contain low numbers of spirochaetes (Moskvitina et al., 1995). Thus, infection of the generative apparatus of male *I. persulcatus* by *B. garinii* may depend on the presence of high numbers of spirochaetes in the tick gut. The preferred transmission of *B. garinii* among tick partners offers an explanation for the predominance of *B. garinii* over *B. afzelii* in field-collected *I. persulcatus* ticks (Alekseev et al., 2010; Korenberg et al., 1997).

Moreover, Alekseev et al. (1999) showed that tick females never transmit *Borrelia* to the *I. persulcatus* males during copulation act. In *I. ricinus* ticks males transmit to the females mostly *B. afzelii*, but the ticks that are more heavily infected by *B. afzelii* do not copulate at all (Alekseev et al., 2010). Dubinina (2000) studied the copulation peculiarities of *Borrelia*-infected/uninfected *I. ricinus* and *I. persulcatus* ticks in laboratory condition. The author reported that *I. ricinus* tick usually copulates on horizontal surfaces, while *I. persulcatus*, on vertical ones. The copulation period of uninfected *I. persulcatus* ticks is 1.3–1.5 times shorter to compare to *I. ricinus*, while borreliae-infection of one or both sexual partners increases the copulation time of *I. persulcatus*.

The *Borrelia*-positive ticks were 35.9% in forest biotopes, 23% in agrarian biocenoses and 36.7% in urbanocenoses. The author found that quite a number of Lyme borreliosis foci in Moldova have been situated in recreation areas where the contact between ticks and humans can be expected to be high (Movila et al., 2006). Similar data exist for other countries (Daniels et al., 1997; Juntila et al., 1999).

4. Vertebrates species specificity

The efficient persistence of the borreliae in endemic areas requires the involvement of reservoir hosts. Potential hosts for ticks are numerous, and more than 300 vertebrate species have been identified as hosts for *I. ricinus*, including small mammals, birds, larger mammals and reptiles. Among these hosts, some act as blood meal sources and as reservoir hosts for pathogens, others as blood meal sources only. Important, that natural host does not seem to develop clinical manifestations of Lyme disease and it is difficult to evaluate the impact of *Borrelia* infection on their health. Minor clinical manifestations may escape medical attention (Gern, 2009).

Halos et al. (2010) reported that the *B. burgdorferi* s.l. infection prevalence was higher on pastures that had a high percentage of shrubs on the perimeter. This result is consistent with the fact that *B. burgdorferi* s.l. reservoir hosts, i.e., rodents and birds, are particularly concentrated in the shrubby vegetation around pastures (Boyard et al., 2008; Vourc'h et al., 2008). The *B. burgdorferi* s.l. infection prevalence also increased in pastures surrounded by forests with low perimeter length/surface area ratios. The lowest theoretical ratio corresponds to a circle; conversely, a high ratio indicated an indented shape with more edge compared to the surface area, which, again, should favor the small vertebrate abundance. This effect was thus in contrast to what we observed on woodland sites, where the prevalence tended to be associated with fragmented forest (Movila, 2008; Movila et al., 2006). Infected ticks found in pastures could have become infected by feeding on infected reservoir hosts located in the pasture itself or by feeding on infected woodland hosts that then imported the ticks into the pasture (Boyard et al., 2007). Halos et al. (2010) hypothesized that a decreased flow of tick hosts between woodlands and pastures could occur when the forest surrounding the pasture has a high perimeter length/surface area ratio, a characteristic which would consequently hinder the infection prevalence in pasture ticks. This mechanism could be mediated by factors that we have not taken into consideration in this study, such as the pasture isolation from woodlands and the lack of connectivity between woodlands and pastures.

4.1 Mammals as reservoirs for *Borrelia* spp.

Only a few mammal species have been identified as reservoirs for *B. burgdorferi* s.l. in Europe. Globally, little information is available on the real significance of most animal hosts as sources for infecting ticks with *B. burgdorferi* s.l. At present, several species of mice, voles, rats and shrews are recognized as reservoirs of *B. burgdorferi* s.l. in Europe (Gern & Humair, 2002). In particular, it was evidenced that the mice *Sylvaemus flavicollis* (Melchior), *Sylvaemus sylvaticus* (Linnaeus), *Apodemus agrarius* (Pallas) and the vole, *Myodes* (=*Clethrionomys*) *glareolus* (Schreber), play key roles in the ecology of Lyme borreliosis as reservoirs for *B. burgdorferi* s.l. in many European countries. Once infected by an infectious tick bite, some reservoir hosts, like *Sylvaemus* mice, have been shown to persistently remain infectious for ticks. Small rodents are frequently parasitized by larval and nymphal *I. ricinus*, and this also contributes to their importance as reservoirs. Less information has been obtained on the roles of other small mammal species in the maintenance cycles of *Borrelia* in nature. Nevertheless, another species of vole *Microtus agrestis* (Linnaeus) in Sweden, and black rats *Rattus rattus* (Linnaeus) and Norway rats *Rattus norvegicus* (Berkenhout) in urbanized environments in Germany and in Madeira, may serve as sources of infection for *I. ricinus* ticks. Similarly, only few data have been collected on *B. burgdorferi* s.l. in shrews (*Sorex minutus* Linnaeus and *Sorrex araneus* Linnaeus and *Neomys fodiens* (Pennant) or in ticks attached on them. Observations in endemic areas of Germany and France showed that edible dormice *Glis glis* (Linnaeus) and garden dormice *Eliomys quercinus* (Linnaeus) are reservoir hosts for *Borrelia*. Other rodent species, like grey squirrels (*Sciurus carolinensis* Gmelin) in the UK and red squirrels *Sciurus vulgaris* (Linnaeus) in Switzerland also contribute to the amplification of *Borrelia* in the tick population. Interestingly, red and grey squirrels are usually very heavily infested with ticks.

In other investigations in Ireland, Germany and Switzerland, it was reported that the European hedgehog (*Erinaceus europaeus* Linnaeus) also perpetuates *B. burgdorferi* s.l. (Rauter & Hartung, 2005). An enzootic transmission cycle of *B. burgdorferi* s.l. involving hedgehogs and another tick vector, *I. hexagonus*, has been observed in an urban environment. This shows that gardens can also represent zones at risk of Lyme borreliosis as further discussed below. Examination of the role of lagomorphs *Lepus europaeus* (Pallas), *Lepus timidus* (Linnaeus) and *Oryctolagus cuniculus* (Linnaeus) in the support of the enzootic cycle of *B. burgdorferi* s.l. has also elucidated their roles as reservoirs (Gern & Humair, 2002).

Assessment of the reservoir competency of large mammals is clearly a difficult task. It necessitates, if xenodiagnosis is applied, capture of the animals and maintenance in a laboratory structure. The consequence of this is that the role of mediumsized and large mammalian species has been studied less and is not yet clearly understood. Red foxes seem to be implicated in the maintenance of borreliae in nature, as described in Germany. However, these animals do not appear to be very potent reservoirs, since spirochaetes were poorly transmitted to ticks feeding on them. According to various reports, ruminants appear to act primarily as sources of blood for ticks. Controversy long surrounded the exact role of large animals, particularly cervids, in the maintenance cycle of *Borrelia* in endemic areas. Currently, most studies seem to indicate that they do not play a role as reservoirs. In fact, studies undertaken in Sweden and in the UK on roe deer *Capreolus capreolus* (Linnaeus), moose *Alces alces* (Linnaeus), red deer *Cervus elaphus* (Linnaeus) and fallow deer *Dama dama* (Linnaeus) suggested that these species do not infect feeding ticks with *B. burgdorferi* s.l. However, according to some recent developments, the possibility exists that they may act as supports for co-feeding transmission of borreliae between infected and uninfected ticks, and therefore may represent amplifying hosts (for review see Gern, 2009).

To date, it was shown that different *Borrelia* genospecies are associated with different vertebrate host. Our data and data of other authors showed that small rodents of the genus *Apodemus* and of the genus *Myodes* as well as red (*S. vulgaris*) and grey squirrels *Sciurus carolinensis* (Gmelin) were usually infected by *B. afzelii* and less frequently by *B. burgdorferi* s.s. and that they transmitted these 2 *Borrelia* species to ticks feeding on them (Gern, 2009; Movila, 2008). As far as less common *Borrelia* species are concerned, like *B. lusitaniae*. Thus, Dsouli et al. (2006) demonstrated the reservoir role of the lizard *Psammodromus algirus* (Linnaeus) for *B. lusitaniae* in Tunisia, Richter & Matuschka (2006) the roles of the common wall lizard *Podarcis muralis* (Laurenti) and sand lizard *Lacerta agilis* Linnaeus in Germany and Amore et al. (2007) reported that *P. muralis* was a reservoir for this *Borrelia* species in Italy.

4.2 Birds as reservoirs for *Borrelia* spp.

When attention was first directed at the role of birds in the ecology of Lyme borreliosis, their role was minimized (Gern, 2009). However, at the beginning of the 1990s, the reservoir role of birds was clarified in Europe, and now it is commonly accepted that some bird species are reservoirs for *B. burgdorferi* s.l. In 1998, 2 studies clearly defined the reservoir role of birds, one on a passerine bird, the blackbird *Turdus merula* (Linnaeus), the other one on a gallinaceous bird species, the pheasant *Phasianus colchicus* (Linnaeus) (Gern & Humair, 2002). Both studies examined the reservoir role of these bird species using xenodiagnosis. Tick xenodiagnosis consists of infecting uninfected ticks - usually larvae - during feeding on the animal suspected to be reservoir host. The fact that some of the same species of *Borrelia* exist both in the northern and in the southern hemisphere is further evidence that birds participate in the natural circulation of *Borrelia* spirochaetes (Poupon et al., 2006). These results and others have evidenced the contribution of birds to the circulation of *Borrelia* in endemic areas. A transmission cycle of *B. burgdorferi* s.l. was discovered in environmental settings other than the biotopes where *I. ricinus* usually live. In fact, it was demonstrated, on a Swedish island, that *B. burgdorferi* spirochaetes could be maintained in seabird colonies among razorbills *Alca torda* (Linnaeus) by an associated tick species, *I. uriae*. The involvement of seabirds and *I. uriae* (in the marine environment) in the transport of infected *Borrelia garinii* between the northern and the southern hemispheres was described. (Comstedt et al., 2009; Gern et al., 1998; Kurtenbach et al., 2006). In this context, it is interesting to mention that in a laboratory study, reactivation of latent *Borrelia*-infection could be induced in passerines experimentally submitted to stressful conditions simulating migration. This implies that during their migration, birds can infect ticks all along their migration route. Bird migration also allows the transfer and establishment of particular *Borrelia* species, as described for *B. lusitaniae*. In fact, birds migrating between south-west Europe/North Africa to north-western Europe have been suggested to be responsible for the transfer of *B. lusitaniae* from

North Africa and south-west Europe, where this *Borrelia* species clearly dominates, to north-west Europe where it is much less frequent (Poupon et al., 2006).

The most commonly parasitized birds are blackbirds and song thrushes, both ground-dwelling birds, which most likely come into contact with *I. ricinus* subadults. Overall, nymphs were more commonly found on birds than were larvae. This result contrasts with those of previous studies involving rodents, in which nymphs feeding on rodents were less abundant than larvae (Hanincová et al., 2003; Movila et al., 2008; Špitalská et al., 2006).

According to classical theory of Kurtenbach et al. (2002) (Fig. 5), *B. afzelii*, *B. garinii* (NT29 ribotype, OspA type 4*), *B. japonica* and *B. bissettii* are resistant to the rodent complement, that makes rodents appropriate reservoir hosts for these genospecies. *B. garinii* (except the abovementioned strains), *B. valaisiana* and *B. turdi* are resistant to the bird complement. *B. burgdorferi* s.s. has an intermediate resistance to both bird and rodent complement and often seem to be infectious to birds and rodents.

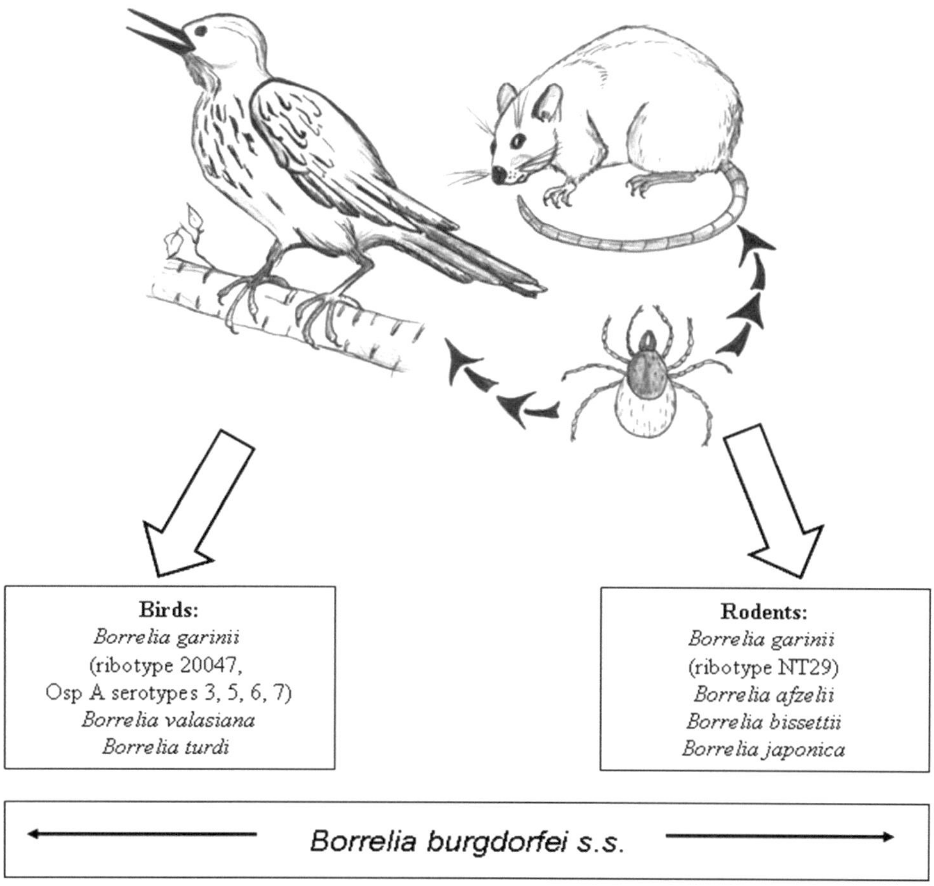

* Margos et al. (2008) proposed a new species *B. bavariensis* as separate from *B. garinii* OspA serotype 4 based on genetic distance and ecological differences.

Fig. 5. Schematic diagram of host specificity of *Borrelia burgdorferi* s.l. (Kurtenbach et al., 2002, with modifications).

A review analysis by Humair (2002) indicated that in Eurasia, *B. garinii* is strongly associated with grounddwelling and sea birds. In Europe, also *B. valaisiana* and *B. burgdorferi* s.s are associated with birds (Derdáková & Lenčaková, 2005). At the same time, Comstedt et al. (2006) demonstrated the presence of five *Borrelia* genospecies (*B. garinii, B. valaisiana, B. afzelii, B. burgdorferi* s.s. and *B. miyamotoi*) in migratory birds in northern Europe. Poupon et al. (2006) found that in Switzerland, *B. valaisiana, B. garinii,* and *B. lusitaniae* were the most frequently found species in ticks collected from migratory birds, with *B. lusitaniae* found in a surprisingly high abundance. In the western Mediterranean Basin, however, a high prevalence of *B. lusitaniae* has been observed in some localities, suggesting that this genospecies has a narrow spectrum of reservoir hosts, restricting its geographical range (de Michelis et al., 2000). *B. lusitaniae* appears to be infrequent in *I. ricinus* in most areas of Europe (Gern et al., 1999), but it has been described as the dominant *Borrelia* species in *I. ricinus* in south-western Europe (de Michelis et al., 2000) and in North Africa (Younsi et al., 2001). Moreover, *B. lusitaniae* was the most frequently detected species after *B. valaisiana* in Moldavian questing *I. ricinus* ticks collected in the "Codri" forest reserve (Movila, 2008). A question for further investigation is whether the dominant *Borrelia* species in birds has shifted from *B. burgdorferi* s.s. to *B. valaisiana* and *B. lusitaniae* during last decades in that area (Movila et al., 2008).

Interestingly, *B. afzelii* was detected in bird-feeding ticks (Comstedt et al., 2006; Kipp et al., 2006; Taragelova et al., 2008), even in engorged larvae (Dubska et al., 2009; Olsen et al., 1995; Poupon et al., 2006), but in relation to other species, the rate was unusually high. Stern et al. (2006) detected *B. afzelii* in only 3 out of 806 bird-feeding ticks from the Greifswalder Oie, using reverse line blot as identification method. The study of Stern et al. (2006) included no robins, accounting for 5 out of 11 *B. afzelii* infections in the present investigation. Dubska et al. (2009) found *B. afzelii* in 13 bird-feeding nymphs and 2 larvae. Although they detected other species more frequently, they suggested that birds may be able to transmit *B. afzelii*.

In Europe, *B. afzelii* occurs in bird-feeding ticks even more frequently than *B. burgdorferi* s.s. (Comstedt et al., 2006; Dubska et al., 2009; Kipp et al., 2006), whereas in North America birds are reservoirs for *B. burgdorferi* s.s. (Jordan et al., 2009; Wright et al., 2006). However, *B. burgdorferi* s.s. seems to be generally rare in many European regions (Burri et al., 2007; Hanincová et al., 2003; Kipp et al., 2006; Smetanova et al., 2007), and consequently this is not necessarily due to a reservoir incompetence of birds for this species in Europe.

There are only a few xenodiagnostic studies on the reservoir competence of birds for certain *Borrelia* species available. Kurtenbach et al. (2002) came to the conclusion that pheasants, a non-passerine species have *B. valaisiana* and *B. garinii* species reservoir competence and no for *B. afzelii*. Another investigation by Ginsberg et al. (2005) states that certain North American passerines, infected with *B. burgdorferi*, show temporal variability in infectiousness to larval ticks, which may be an explanation for different prevalence rates of European genospecies in the literature. This could indicate that the birds may be infected with *B. afzelii*, but transovarial transmission of *B. afzelii* and co-feeding with *B. afzelii*-carrying nymphs may also explain these findings.

There are 3 mechanisms of the birds' role in spreading *Borrelia*-infected ticks:

1. Passive transport of previously infected nymphs and transovarially infected larvae may occur.

2. Infected migratory birds may infect the ticks, which are then dropped off in a new location. In support of this mechanism, Gylfe et al. (2000) found a reactivation of *B. garinii* infection in experimentally infected *Turdus iliacus* Linnaeus during migratory restlessness, indicating an increased risk of transmitting *Borrelia* sp. to the tick vector during migration. If the migratory birds are chronic carriers of tick-borne diseases, then they may continue to transfer them to ticks that parasitize them after arrival. Sampling of blood or tissue from the birds would provide more information of this issue.
3. The tick vectors may transfer *Borrelia* species between each other through co-feeding while being transported (Randolph et al., 1998; Dubinina & Alekseev, 2003).

5. Conclusion

The description of the various *Borrelia* species in ticks has opened an entire new field of research in the ecology of Lyme borreliosis. It seems prudent to review the importance of the different types of associations between *Borrelia* species, tick vectors, and vertebrate hosts in various geographic areas.

Host specialization is an important factor in vector-borne disease, and different pathogens show varying levels and patterns of host specialization, which may impact the spread of pathogens. Lyme borreliosis group of spirochaetes, *B. garinii* and *B. valaisiana* are transmitted by avian species while *B. afzelii* is associated with rodents and certain insectivore species. *B. burgdorferi* s.s. is a generalist species, known to infect both rodent and avian species, as well as other hosts. The diversity in host specialisms in the Lyme borreliosis group of spirochaetes makes this an ideal system to examine the interplay between the ecology of the host and the epidemiology of the bacteria. As ticks do not move over large distances independently, the spread of *Borrelia* spp. spirochaetes is likely to be linked to the migration of their hosts. Species that are maintained by rodents are therefore predicted to show more limited migration than those associated with birds. In addition to being of public health importance, the delineation and monitoring of the geographic ranges of the different Lyme borreliosis species also provides an opportunity to examine in more general terms the role of host ecology in the epidemiology of vectored zoonoses.

Clearly, additional field studies are needed of *Borrelia* host specificities, keeping in mind particularly the newly described *Borrelia* species and the great subtype diversity hidden in most *Borrelia* species, as well as the geographic diversity of local ecosystems. Future studies in Lyme borreliosis ecology seeking to identify the *Borrelia* spirochaetes in both ticks and reservoir hosts in various endemic areas are strongly encouraged. Those studies are extremely important for the determination of the complete spectrum of *Borrelia* species involved in human Lyme disease worldwide with its unknown, rare, and unusual clinical manifestation.

6. Acknowledgment

We indebted to Mr. Igor Babic (InTech Open Access Publisher) and Mr. Alexandr Morozov (Institute of Zoology, Moldova) for rendered assistance in this chapter preparation. We acknowledge the perfect original images of Mrs. Anna Movila. The authors thank Moldova Academy of Science for financial support.

7. References

Alekseev, A.N. 1984. On the specificity of arthropods as the vectors of the agents of transmissive diseases and the type of symbiotic relations between them and pathogens. *Parazitological Revue*, Vol.32, (May 1984), pp. 43–60, ISSN 0370-1794, Leningrad (In Russian, English Resume)

Alekseev, A.N. & Kondrashova, Z.N. (1985). *Organism of arthropods as environment for pathogens*. Academy of Sciences USSR, Sverdlovsk (In Russian, English Resume)

Alekseev, A.N. (1992). Ecology of tick-borne encephalitis virus: part of Ixodidae tick males in its circulation. *Ecological parasitology*, Vol.1, No.1, (March 1992), pp. 48–58, ISSN 0869-396X

Alekseev, A.N. & Dubinina, E.V. (1994). Symbiotic relationships in the complex carrier-pathogen system. *Doklady Akademii Nauk*, Vol.338, No.2, (September 1994), pp. 259–261, ISSN 0869-5652

Alekseev, A.N. & Dubinina, H.V. (2006). Evidence that tick attachment to the human body isn't random. *Acarina*, Vol.14, No.2, (December 2006), pp. 203–208, ISSN 0132-8077

Alekseev, A.N.; Dubinina, H.V.; Antykova, L.P.; Dzhivanyan, T.I.; Rijpkema, S.G.; Kruif, N.V. & Cinco, M. (1998). Tick-borne borrelioses pathogen identification in *Ixodes* ticks (Acarina, Ixodidae) collected in St. Petersburg and Kaliningrad Baltic regions of Russia. *Journal of Medical Entomology*, Vol.35, No.2, (March 1998), pp. 136–142, ISSN 0022-2585

Alekseev, A.N.; Dubinina, H.V. & Jushkova, O.V. (2010). *Influence of Anthropogenic Pressure on the System "Tick-tick-borne Pathogens"*, Pensoft Pub, ISBN 9789546425652, Sofia - Moscow - St. Petersburg

Alekseev, A.N.; Dubinina, H.V.; Rijpkema, S.G.T. & Schouls, L.M. (1999). Sexual transmission of *Borrelia garinii* by male *Ixodes persulcatus* ticks (Acari, Ixodidae). *Experimental and Applied Acarology*, Vol.23, No.2, (February 1999), pp. 165–169, ISSN 0168-8162

Alekseev, A.N.; Jensen, P.M.; Dubinina, H.V.; Smirnova, L.A.; Makrouchina, N.A. & Zharkov, S.D. (2000). Peculiarities of behaviour of taiga (*Ixodes persulcatus*) and sheep (*Ixodes ricinus*) ticks (Acarina: Ixodidae) determined by different methods. *Folia Parasitologica*, Vol.47, No.2, (March 2000), pp. 147–153, ISSN 0015-5683

Anderson, J.F.; Barthold, S.W. & Magnarelli, L.A. (1990). Infectious but nonpathogenic isolate of *Borrelia burgdorferi*. *Journal of Clinical Microbiology*, Vol.28, No.12, (December 1995), pp. 2693–2699, ISSN 0095-1137

Anguita, J.; Ramamoorthi, N.; Hovius, J.W.; Das, S.; Thomas, V.; Persinski, R.; Conze, D.; Askenase, P.W.; Rincón, M.; Cantor, F.S. & Fikrig, E. (2002). Salp15, an *Ixodes scapularis* salivary gland protein, inhibits CD4(+) T cell activation. *Immunity*, Vol.16, Issue.6, (June 2002), pp. 849–859, ISSN 1074-7613

Amore, G.; Tomassone, L.; Grego, E.; Ragagli, C.; Bertolotti, L.; Nebbia, P.; Rosati, S. & Mannelli, A. (2007). *Borrelia lusitaniae* in immature *Ixodes ricinus* (Acari: Ixodidae) feeding on common wall lizards in Tuscany, Central Italy. *Journal of Medical Entomology*, Vol.44, No.2, (February 2007), pp. 303–307, ISSN 0022-2585

Babenko, L.V. (1985). Sexual composition of the population. Sites of sexes' encounters and the occurrence of inseminated active unfed females, In: *Taiga tick Ixodes persulcatus Schulze (Acarina, Ixodidae). Morphology, Systematics, Ecology, Medical importance*, N.A. Filippova, (Ed.), 245-248, Nauka, Leningrad, USSR (In Russian)

Baranton, G.; Postic, D.; Saint Girons, I.; Boerlin, P.; Piffaretti, J.C.; Assous, M. & Grimont, P.A. (1992). Delineation of *Borrelia burgdorferi* sensu stricto, *Borrelia garinii* sp. nov., and group VS461 associated with Lyme borreliosis. *International Journal of Systematic Bacteriology*, Vol.42, No.3, (July 1992), pp. 378-383, ISSN 0020-7713

Boyard, C.; Barnouin, J.; Gasqui, P. & Vourc'h, G. (2007). Local environmental factors characterizing *Ixodes ricinus* nymph abundance in grazed permanent pastures for cattle. *Parasitology*, Vol.134, No.7, (July 2007), pp. 987-994, ISSN 0031-1820

Boyard, C.; Vourc'h, G. & Barnouin, J. (2008). The relationships between *Ixodes ricinus* and small mammal species at the woodland-pasture interface. *Experimental and Applied Acarology*, Vol.44, No.1, (January 2008), pp. 61-76, ISSN 0168-8162

Burri, C.; Cadenas, F.M.; Douet, V.; Moret, J. & Gern, L. (2007). *Ixodes ricinus* density and infection prevalence of *Borrelia burgdorferi* sensu lato along a North-facing altitudinal gradient in the Rhone Valley (Switzerland). *Vector-Borne and Zoonotic Diseases*, Vol.7, No.1, (April 2006), pp. 50-58, ISSN 1530-3667

Canica, M.M.; Nato, F.; du Merle, L.; Mazie, J.C.; Baranton, G. & Postic, D. (1993). Monoclonal antibodies for identification of *Borrelia afzelii* sp. nov. associated with late cutaneous manifestations of Lyme borreliosis. *Scandinavian Journal of Infectious Diseases*, Vol.25, No.4, (December 1993), pp. 441-448, ISSN 0036-5548

Chu, C.Y.; Liu, W.; Juany, B.G.; Wang, D.M.; Juany, W.J.; Zhao, Q.M.; Zhang, P.H.; Wang, Z.X.; Tang, G.P.; Yang H. & Cao, W.C. (2008). Novel genospecies of *Borrelia burgdorferi* sensu lato from rodents and ticks in southwestern China. *Journal of Clinical Microbiology*, Vol.46, No.9, (September 2008), pp. 3130-3133, ISSN 0095-1137

Chunikhin, S.P.; Stefutkina, L.F., Korolev, M.B., Reshetnikov, I.A. & Khozinskaya G.A. (1983). Sexual transmission of tick-borne encephalitis virus in ixodids (Ixodidae). *Parazitologiya*, Vol.17, No.3, (June 1983), pp. 214-217, ISSN 0031-1847 (In Russian)

Crippa, M.; Rais, O. & Gern, L. (2002). Investigations on the mode and dynamics of transmission and infectivity of *Borrelia burgdorferi* sensu stricto and *Borrelia afzelii* in *Ixodes ricinus* ticks. *Vector-Borne and Zoonotic Diseases*, Vol.2, No.1, (July 2004), pp. 3-9, ISSN 1530-3667

Comstedt, P.; Bergström, S.; Olsén, B.; Garpmo, U.; Marjavaara, L.; Mejlon, H.; Barbour A.G. & Bunikis, J. (2006) Migratory passerine birds as reservoirs of Lyme borreliosis in Europe. *Emerging Infectious Diseases*, Vol.12, No.7, (July 2006), pp. 1087-1095, ISSN 1080-6040

Comstedt, P.; Asokliene, L.; Eliasson, I.; Olsen, B.; Wallensten, A.; Bunikis, J. & Bergström, S. (2009). Complex population structure of Lyme borreliosis group spirochete Borrelia garinii in subarctic Eurasia. *PLoS One*, Vol.9, No.6, (June 2009), e5841, ISSN 1932-6203

de Michelis, S.; Sewell, H.S.; Collares-Pereira, M.; Santos-Reis, M.; Schouls, L.M.; Benes, V.; Holmes, E.C. & Kurtenbach, K. (2000). Genetic diversity of *Borrelia burgdorferi* sensu lato in ticks from mainland Portugal. *Journal of Clinical Microbiology*, Vol.38, No.6, (June 2000), pp. 2128-2133, ISSN 0095-1137

Daniel, M.; Danielova, V.; Kriz, B.; Jirsa, A. & Nozicka J. (2003). Shift of the tick *Ixodes ricinus* and tick-borne encephalitis to higher altitudes in central Europe. *European*

Journal of Clinical Microbiology and Infectious Diseases, Vol.22, No.5, (May 2003), pp. 327-328, ISSN 0934-9723

Daniels, T.J.; Falco, R.C.; Schwartz, I.; Varde, S. & Robbins, R.G. (1997). Deer ticks (*Ixodes scapularis*) and the agents of Lyme disease and human granulocytic ehrlichiosis in a New York City park. *Emerging Infectious Diseases*, Vol.3, No.3, (July-September 1997), pp. 353-355, ISSN 1080-6040

Derdáková, M. & Lenčaková, D. (2005). Association of genetic variability within the *Borrelia burgdorferi* sensu lato with the ecology, epidemiology of Lyme borreliosis in Europe. *Annals of Agricultural and Environmental Medicine*, Vol.12, No.2, (June 2005), pp. 165-172, ISSN 1232-1966

Dsouli, N.; Younsi-Kabachii, H.; Postic, D.; Nouira, S.; Gern, L. & Bouattour, A. (2006). Reservoir role of the lizard, *Psammodromus algirus*, in the transmission cycle of *Borrelia burgdorferi* sensu lato (Spirochaetacea) in Tunisia. *Journal of Medical Entomology*, Vol.43, No.4, (April 2006), pp. 737-742, ISSN 0022-2585

Du, Y.; Tou, X.; Wu, X. & Qien, Z.H. (1990). Dissemination and transovarial transmission of *Borrelia burgdorferi* in *Ixodes persulcatus* (Acari: Ixodidae). *Chinese Journal of Vector Biology and Control*, Vol.1, No.6, (December 1990), pp 367-369, ISSN 1003-4692 (In Chinese)

Dubinina, H.V. (2000). Some peculiarities of the mating behaviour in *Ixodes persulcatus* and *Ixodes ricinus* ticks (Acarina, Ixodidae): differences in a sexual transmission of the species of *Borrelia*. *Acarina*, Vol.8, No.2, (July 2000), pp. 125-131, ISSN 0132-8077

Dubinina, H.V. & Alekseev, A.N. (2003). The role of migratory passerine birds in pathogen exchange between cofeeding *Ixodes ricinus* ticks (Acarina, Ixodidae). *Acarina*, Vol.11, No.1, (November 2003), pp. 99-104, ISSN 0132-8077

Dubinina, E.V. & Makurshina, N.A. (1997). The characteristics of the circadian rhythm in the activities of *Ixodes ricinus* ticks on the Kurskaia Kosa (Kaliningrad Province). *Meditsinskaia Parazitologiia (Moscow)*, No.3, (July-September 1997), pp. 42-44, ISSN 0025-8326 (In Russian)

Dubska, L.; Literak, I.; Kocianova, E.; Taragelova, V. & Sychra, O. (2009). Differential role of passerine birds in distribution of *Borrelia* spirochaetes, based on data from ticks collected from birds during the post breeding migration period in Central Europe. *Applied and Environmental Microbiology*, Vol.75, No.3, (February 2009), pp. 596-602, ISSN 0099-2240

Eisen, L. & Lane, R.S. (2002). Vectors of *Borrelia burgdorferi* sensu lato, In: *Lyme Borreliosis: Biology, Epidemiology and Control*, J.S. Gray, O.; Kahl, R.S. Lane & G. Stanek, (Eds.), pp 91-115, CAB International, ISBN 9780851996325, Wallingford

Falco, R.C.; Fish, D. & Piesman, J. (1996). Duration of tick bites in a Lyme disease-endemic area. *American Journal of Epidemiology*, Vol.143, No.2, (January 1996), pp. 187-192, ISSN 0002-9262

Filippova, N.A. (1977). *Ixodid ticks of the subfamily Ixodinae*, Nauka, Leningrad, USSR

Fukunaga, M.; Hamase, A.; Okada, K.; Inoue, H.; Tsuruta, Y.; Miyamoto, K. & Nakao, M. (1996a). Characterization of spirochaetes isolated from ticks (*Ixodes tanuki*, *Ixodes turdus*, and *Ixodes columnae*) and comparison of the sequences with those of *Borrelia burgdorferi* sensu lato strains. *Applied and Environmental Microbiology*, Vol.62, No.7, (July 1996), pp. 2338-2344, ISSN 0099-2240

Fukunaga, M.; Hamase, A.; Okada, K. & Nakao, M. (1996b). *Borrelia tanukii* sp. nov. and *Borrelia turdae* sp. nov. found from ixodid ticks in Japan: rapid species identification by 16S rRNA gene-targeted PCR analysis. *Microbiology and Immunology*, Vol.40, No.11, (November 1996), pp. 877–881, ISSN 0385-5600

Gaber, M.S.; Khalil, G.M. & Hoogstraal, H. (1982). *Borrelia crocidurae*: venereal transfer in Egyptian *Ornithodorus erraticus* ticks. *Experimental Parasitology*, Vol.54, No.2, (October 1982), pp. 182–184, ISSN 0014-4894

Gaber, M.S.; Khalil, G.M.; Hoogstraal, H. & Aboul-Nasr, A.E. (1984). *Borrelia crocidurae* localization and transmission in *Ornithodoros erraticus* and *O. savignyi*. Parasitology Vol.88, No.3, (June 1984), pp. 403–413, ISSN 0031-1820

Garg, R.; Juncadella, I.J.; Ramamoorthi, N.; Ashish; Ananthanarayanan, S.K.; Thomas, V.; Rincón, M.; Krueger, J.K.; Fikrig, E.; Yengo, Ch.M. & Anguita, J. (2006). Cutting edge: CD4 is the receptor for the tick saliva immunosuppressor, Salp15. *The Journal of Immunology*, Vol.177, No.10, (November 2006), pp. 6579-6583, ISSN 1550-6606

Gern, L. (2009). Life cycle of *Borrelia burgdorferi* sensu lato and transmission to humans. In: *Current problems of Dermatology*, D. Lipsker & J. Benoît, (Eds.), pp. 18–30, Karger, ISBN 9783805591140, Basel

Gern, L.; Estrada-Peña, A.; Frandsen, F.; Gray, J.S.; Jaenson, T.G.; Jongejan, F.; Kahl, O.; Korenberg, E.; Mehl, R. & Nuttall, P.A. (1998). European reservoir hosts of *Borrelia burgdorferi* sensu lato. *Zentralblatt für Bakteriologie*, Vol.287, No.3, (March 1998), pp. 196-204, ISSN 0934-8840

Gern, L.; Hu, C.M.; Kocianova, E.; Vyrostekova, V. & Rehacek, J. (1999). Genetic diversity of *Borrelia burgdorferi* sensu lato isolates obtained from *Ixodes ricinus* ticks collected in Slovakia. *European Journal of Epidemiology*, Vol.15, No.7, (August 1999), pp. 665–669, ISSN 0393-2990

Gern, L. & Humair, P.F. (2002). Ecology of *Borrelia burgdorferi* sensu lato in Europe. In: *Lyme Borreliosis: Biology, Epidemiology and Control*, J.S. Gray, O. Kahl, R.S. Lane, & G. Stanek, (Eds), pp 149–174, CAB International, ISBN 9780851996325, Wallingford

Ginsberg, H.S.; Buckley, P.A.; Balmforth, M.G.; Zhioua, E.; Mitra, S., & Buckley, F.G. (2005). Reservoir competence of native North American birds for the Lyme disease spirochete, *Borrelia burgdorferi*. *Journal of Medical Entomology*, Vol.42, No.3, (May 2005), pp. 445–449, ISSN 0022-2585

Gorelova, N.B.; Korenberg, E.I.; Kovalevskiĭ, Iu.V.; Postic, D. & Baranton, G. (1996). The isolation of *Borrelia* from the tick *Ixodes trianguliceps* (Ixodidae) and the possible significance of this species in the epizootiology of ixodid tick-borne borrelioses. *Parazitologiya.*, Vol.30, No.1, (January-February 1996), pp.13–18, ISSN 0031-1847

Gylfe, A.; Bergström, S.; Lundström, J. & Olsen, B. (2000). Reactivation of *Borrelia* infection in birds. *Nature*, Vol.403, (February 2000), pp. 724–725, ISSN 0028-0836

Halos, L.; Bord, S.; Cotté, V.; Gasqui, P.; Abrial, D.; Barnouin, J.; Boulouis, H.J.; Vayssier-Taussat, M. & Vourc'h, G. (2010). Ecological factors characterizing the prevalence of bacterial tick-borne pathogens in *Ixodes ricinus* ticks in pastures and woodlands. *Applied and Environmental Microbiology*, Vol.76, No.13, (July 2010), pp. 4413–4420, ISSN 0099-2240

Hanincová, K.; Schäfer, S.M.; Etti, S.; Sewell, H.S.; Taragelová, V.; Ziak, D.; Labuda, M. & Kurtenbach, K. (2003). Association of *Borrelia afzelii* with rodents in Europe. *Parasitology*, Vol.126, No.1, (January 2003), pp. 11–20, ISSN 0031-1820

Herrmann, C. & Gern, L. 2010. Survival of *Ixodes ricinus* (Acari: Ixodidae) under challenging conditions of temperature and humidity is influenced by Borrelia burgdorferi sensu lato infection. *Journal of Medical Entomology*, Vol.47, No.6, (November 2010), pp. 1196–1204, ISSN 0022-2585

Hovius, J.W.R.; de Jong, M.A.W.P.; den Dunnen, J.; Litjens, M.; Fikring, E.; van der Poll, T.; Ringhuis, S.I. & Geijtenbeek T.B.H. 2008. Salp15 binding to DC-SIGN inhibits cytokine expression by impairing both nucleosome remodeling and mRNA stabilizations. PLOS Pathogogens, Vol.4, Issue2, (February 2008), e31, ISSN 1553-7366

Humair, P.-F. (2002). Birds and *Borrelia*. *International Journal of Medical Microbiology*, Vol.291, Suppl.33, (June 2002), pp. 70–74, ISSN 1438-4221

Jaenson, T.G.; Tälleklint, L.; Lundqvist, L.; Olsen, B.; Chirico, J. & Mejlon, H. (1994). Geographical distribution, host associations, and vector roles of ticks (Acari: Ixodidae, Argasidae) in Sweden. *Journal of Medical Entomology*, Vol.31, No.2, (March 1994), pp. 240–256, ISSN 0022-2585

Jordan, B.E.; Onks, K.R.; Hamilton, S.W.; Hayslette, S.E. & Wright, S.M. (2009). Detection of *Borrelia burgdorferi* and *Borrelia lonestari* in birds in Tennessee. *Journal of Medical Entomology*, No.46, Vol.1, (January 2009), pp. 131–138, ISSN 0022-2585

Juntila, J.; Peltomaa, M.; Soini, H.; Marjamaki, M. & Viljanen, K.M. (1999). Prevalence of *Borrelia burgdorferi* in *Ixodes ricinus* ticks in urban recreational areas of Helsinki. *Journal of Clinical Microbiology*, Vol.37, No.5, (May 1999), pp. 1361–1365, ISSN 0095-1137

Kahl, O.; Janetzki-Mittmann, C.; Gray, J.S.; Jonas, R.; Stein, J. & de Boer, R. (1998). Risk of infection with *Borrelia burgdorferi* sensu lato for a host in relation to the duration of nymphal *Ixodes ricinus* feeding and the method of tick removal. *Zentralblatt fur Bakteriologie Microbiologie und Hygiene*, Vol.287, No.1-2, (January 1998), pp. 41–52, ISSN 0934-8840.

Kawabata, H.; Masuzawa, T. & Yanagihara, Y. (1993). Genomic analysis of *Borrelia japonica* sp. nov. isolated from *Ixodes ovatus* in Japan. *Microbiology and Immunology*, Vol.37, No.11, (November 1993), pp. 843–848, ISSN 0385-5600

Kipp, S.; Goedecke, A.; Dorn, W.; Wilske, B. &, Fingerle, V. (2006). Role of birds in Thuringia, Germany, in the natural cycle of *Borrelia burgdorferi* sensu lato, the Lyme disease spirochaete. *International Journal of Medical Microbiology*, Vol.296, Suppl.1, (May 2006), pp. 125–128, ISSN 1438-4221

Korenberg, E.I.; Gorelova, N.B.; Postic, D.; Kovalevsky, Yu.V.; Baranton, G. & Vorobyeva, N.N. (1997). Reservoir hosts and vectors of *Borrelia*, causative agents of ixodid tick-borne borrelioses in Russia. *Journal of Microbiology Epidemiology and Immunobiology*, Vol.6, (November-December 1997), pp. 36–38, ISSN 0372-9311 (In Russian)

Korenberg, E.I.; Nefedova, V.V.; Romanenko, V.N. & Gorelova, N.B. The tick *Ixodes pavlovskyi* as a host of spirochetes pathogenic for humans and its possible role in the epizootiology and epidemiology of borrelioses. *Vector Borne and Zoonotic Diseases*, Vol.10, No.5, (June 2010), pp. 453-458, ISSN 1530-3667

Kovalevskii, Y.V. & Korenberg, E.I. (1995). Differences in *Borrelia* infections in adult *Ixodes persulcatus* and *Ixodes ricinus* ticks (Acari: Ixodidae) in populations of north-western Russia. *Experimental and Applied Acarology*, Vol.19, No.1, (January 1995), pp. 19–29, ISSN 0168-8162

Kurtenbach, K.; Peacey, M.; Rijpkema, S.G.; Hoodless, A.N.; Nuttall, P.A. & Randolph, S.E. (1998). Differential transmission of the genospecies of *Borrelia burgdorferi* sensu lato by game birds and small rodents in England. *Applied and Environmental Microbiology*, Vol.64, No.4, (April 1998), pp. 1169–1174, ISSN 0099-2240

Kurtenbach, K.; De Michelis, S.; Etti, S.; Schäfer, S.M.; Sewell, H.S.; Brade, V. & Kraiczy, P. (2002). Host association of *Borrelia burgdorferi* sensu lato the key role of host complement. *Trends in Microbiology*, Vol.10, No.2, (February, 2002), pp. 74–79, ISSN 0966-842X

Kurtenbach, K.; Hanincová, K.; Tsao, J.I.; Margos, G.; Fish, D. & Ogden, N.H. (2006). Fundamental processes in the evolutionary ecology of Lyme borreliosis. *Nature Reviews Microbiology*, Vol.4, No.9, (September 2006), pp. 660–669, ISSN 1740-1526

Lane, R.S. & Burgdorfer, W. (1987). Transovarial and Transstadial Passage of *Borrelia burgdorferi* in the Western Black-Legged Tick, *Ixodes pacificus* (Acari: Ixodidae). *American Journal of Tropical Medicine and Hygiene*, Vol.37, No.1, (July. 1987), pp. 188–192, ISSN 0002-9637

Le Fleche, A.; Postic, D.; Girardet, K.; Péter O. & Baranton, G. (1997). Characterization of *Borrelia lusitaniae* sp. nov. by 16S ribosomal DNA sequence analysis. *International Journal of Systematic Bacteriology*, Vol.47, No.4, (October 1997), pp. 921–925, ISSN 0020-7713

Lefcort, H. & Durden, L.A. (1996). The effect of infection with Lyme disease spirochaetes (*Borrelia burgdorferi*) on the phototaxis, activity, and questing height of the tick vector *Ixodes scapularis*. *Parasitology*, Vol.113, No.2, (August 1996), pp. 97–103, ISSN 0031-1820.

Lees, A.D. & Milne, A. (1951). The seasonal and diurnal activities of individual sheep ticks (*Ixodes ricinus* L.). *Parasitology*, Vol.41, No.3-4, (December 1951), pp. 189–208, ISSN 0031-1820

Marconi, R.T.; Liveris, D. & Schwartz, I. (1995). Identification of novel insertion elements, restriction fragment length polymorphism patterns, and discontinuous 23S rRNA in Lyme disease spirochaetes: phylogenetic analyses of rRNA genes and their intergenic spacers in *Borrelia japonica* sp. nov. and genomic group 21038 (*Borrelia andersonii* sp.nov.) isolates. *Journal of Clinical Microbiology*, Vol.33, No.9, (September 1995), pp. 2427–2434, ISSN 0095-1137

Margos, G.; Gatewood, A.G.; Aanensen, D.M.; Hanincova, K.; Terekhova, D.; Vollmer, S.A.; Cornet, M.; Piesman, J.; Donaghy, M.; Bormane, A.; Hurn, M.A.; Feil, E.J.; Fish, D.; Casjens, S.; Wormser, G.P.; Schwartz, I. & Kurtenbach, K. (2008). MLST of housekeeping genes captures geographic population structure and suggests a European origin of *Borrelia burgdorferi*. *Proceedings of the National Academy of Sciences of the United States of America*, Vol.105, No.25, (June 2008), pp. 8730–8735, ISSN 0027-8424

Margos, G.; Vollmer, S.A.; Kornet, M.; Garnier, M.; Fingerle, V.; Wilske, B.; Bormane, A.; Vitorino, L.; Collares-Pereira, M.; Drancourt, M. & Kurtenbach, K. (2009). A new *Borrelia* species defined by multilocus sequence analysis of housekeeping genes.

Applied and Environmental Microbiology, Vol.75, No.16, (August 2009), pp. 5410-5416, ISSN 0099-2240

Margos, G.; Hojgaard, A.; Lane, R.S.; Cornet, M.; Fingerle, V.; Rudenko, N.; Ogden, N.; Aanensen, D.M.; Fish D. & Piesman, J. (2010). Multilocus sequence analysis of *Borrelia bissettii* strains from North America reveals a new *Borrelia* species, *Borrelia kurtenbachii*. *Ticks and Tick-borne Diseases*, Vol.1, No.4, (December 2010), pp. 151-158, ISSN 1877-959X

Margos, G.; Vollmer, S.A.; Ogden, N.H. & Fish D. (2011). Population genetics, taxonomy, phylogeny and evolution of *Borrelia burgdorferi* sensu lato. *Infection, Genetics and Evolution*, doi:10.1016/j.meegid.2011.07.022, ISSN 1567-1348

Masuzawa, T.; Takada, N.; Kudeken, M.; Fukui, T.; Yano, Y.; Ishiguro, F.; Kawamura, Y.; Imai Y. & Ezaki, T. (2001). *Borrelia sinica* sp. nov., a Lyme disease-related *Borrelia* species isolated in China. *International Journal of Systematic and Evolutionary Microbiology*, Vol.51, No.5, (September 2001), pp. 1817-1824, ISSN 1466-5026

Mátlová, L.; Halouzka, J.; Juricova, Z. & Hubalek, Z. (1996). Comparative experimental infection of *Ixodes ricinus* and *Dermacentor reticulatus* (Acari: Ixodidae) with *Borrelia burgdorferi* sensu lato. *Folia Parasitologica*, Vol.43, No.2, (March 1996), pp. 159-160, ISSN 0015-5683

Meiners, T.; Hammer, B.; Göbel, U.B. & Kahl, O. (2006). Determining the tick scutal index allows assessment of tick feeding duration and estimation of infection risk with *Borrelia burgdorferi* sensu lato in a person bitten by an *Ixodes ricinus* nymph. *International Journal of Medical Microbiology*, Vol.296, Suppl.40, (May 2006), pp. 103-107, ISSN 1438-4221

Morshed, M.G.; Scott, J.D.; Fernando, K.; Beati, L.; Mazerolle, D.F.; Geddes, G. & Durden, L.A. (2005). Migratory songbirds disperse ticks across Canada, and first isolation of the Lyme disease spirochete, *Borrelia burgdorferi*, from the avian tick, *Ixodes auritulus*. *Journal of Parasitology*, Vol.91, No.4, (August 2005), pp. 780-790, ISSN 0022-3395

Moskvitina, G.G.; Korenberg, E.I.; Spielman, A. & Schhyogolova, T.V. (1995). On frequencies of generalized infection in unfed adult ticks of the genus *Ixodes* in Russian and American foci of the borrelioses. *Parazitologiya*, Vol.29, No.5, (September-October 1995), pp. 353-360, ISSN 0031-1847 (In Russian)

Movila, A. (2008). Genetic diversity of ixodid ticks *Ixodes ricinus* (L.) and tick-borne pathogens in foci of the Republic of Moldova. PhD-thesis summary, In: *www.cnaa.md*, September 2008, Available from www.cnaa.md/thesis/11675/

Movila, A.; Uspenskaia, I.; Toderas, I.; Melnic, V. & Conovalov, J. (2006) Prevalence of *Borrelia burgdorferi* sensu lato and *Coxiella burnetti* in ticks collected in different biocenoses in the Republic of Moldova. *International Journal of Medical Microbiology*, Vol.296, Suppl.1, (May 2006), pp. 172-176, ISSN 1438-4221

Movila, A.; Gatewood, A.; Toderas, I.; Duca, M.; Papero, M.; Uspenskaia, I.; Conovalov, Ju. & Fish, D. (2008). Prevalence of *Borrelia burgdorferi* sensu lato in *Ixodes ricinus* and *I. lividus* ticks collected from wild birds in the Republic of Moldova. *International Journal of Medical Microbiology*, Vol.298, Suppl.1, (September 2008), pp. 149-153, ISSN 1438-4221

Nakao, M. & Miyamoto, K. (1992). Negative finding in detection of transovarial transmission of *Borrelia burgdorferi* in Japanese ixodid ticks, *Ixodes persulcatus* and

Ixodes ovatus. Japanese Journal of Sanitary Zoology, Vol.43, pp. 343-345, ISSN 0424-7086

Nefedova, V.V.; Korenberg, E.I.; Gorelova, N.B. & Kovalevskii, Y.V. (2004). Studies on the transovarial transmission of *Borrelia burgdorferi* sensu lato in the taiga tick *Ixodes persulcatus. Folia Parasitologica*, Vol.51, No.1, (March 2004), pp. 67-71, ISSN 0015-5683

Okulova, N.M. (1978). The vertical and horizontal movement of Ixodidae ticks in the forest in depending from the temperature and air humidity. *Russian Journal of Ecology*, Vol.2, pp. 44-48, ISSN 1067-4136 (In Russian)

Olsen, B.; Jaenson, T. & Bergstrom, S. (1995). Prevalence of *Borrelia burgdorferi* sensu lato-infected ticks on migrating birds. *Applied and Environmental Microbiology*, Vol.61, No.8, (August 1995), pp. 3082-3087, ISSN 0099-2240

Pal, U.; Yang, X.; Chen, M.; Bockenstedt, L.K.; Anderson, J.F.; Flavell, R.A.; Norgard, M.V. & Fikrig, E. (2004). OspC facilitates *Borrelia burgdorferi* invasion of *Ixodes scapularis* salivary glands. *The Journal of Clinical Investigation*, Vol.113, No.2, (January 2004), pp. 220-230, ISSN 0021-9738

Peavey, C.A. & Lane, R.S. (1995). Transmission of *Borrelia burgdorferi* by *Ixodes pacificus* nymphs and reservoir competence of deer mice (*Peromyscus maniculatus*) infected by tick-bite. *Journal of Parasitology*, Vol.81, No.4, (April 1995), pp. 175-178, ISSN 0022-3395

Piesman, J. (2002). Ecology of *Borrelia burgdorferi* sensu lato in Northamerica, In: *Lyme Borreliosis: Biology, Epidemiology and Control*, J.S. Gray, O. Kahl, R.S. Lane & G. Stanek, (Eds.), pp 223-249, CAB International, ISBN 9780851996325, Wallingford

Piesman, J. & Spielman, A. (1980). Human babesiosis on Nantucket Island: prevalence of Babesia microti in ticks. *American Journal of Tropical Medicine and Hygiene*, Vol.29, No.5, (September 1995), pp. 742-746, ISSN 0002-9637

Piesman, J.; Mather, J.M.; Sinsky, R.J. & Spielman, A. (1987). Duration of tick attachment and *Borrelia burgdorferi* transmission. *Journal of Clinical Microbiology*, Vol.25, No.3, (March 1987), pp. 557-558, ISSN 0095-1137

Piesman, J.; Maupin, G.O.; Campos, E.G. & Happ, C.M. (1991). Duration of adult female *Ixodes dammini* attachment and transmission of *Borrelia burgdorferi*, with description of a needle aspiration isolation method. *Journal of Infectious Diseases*, Vol.163, No.4, (April 1991), pp. 895-897, ISSN 0022-1899

Postic, D.; Ras, N.M.; Lane, R.S.; Hendson, M. & Baranton, G. (1998). Expanded diversity among Californian borrelia isolates and description of *Borrelia bissettii* sp. nov. (formerly *Borrelia* group DN127). *Journal of Clinical Microbiology*, Vol.36, No.12, (December 1998), pp. 3497-3504, ISSN 0095-1137

Postic, D.; Garnier, M. & Baranton, G. (2007). Multilocus sequence analysis of atypical *Borrelia burgdorferi* sensu lato isolates - description of *Borrelia californiensis* sp. nov., and genomospecies 1 and 2. *International Journal of Medical Microbiology*, Vol.297, No.4, (July 2007), pp. 263-271, ISSN 1438-4221

Poupon, M.A.; Lommano, E.; Humair, P.F.; Douet, V.; Rais, O.; Schaad, M.; Jenni, L. & Gern, L. (2006). Prevalence of *Borrelia burgdorferi* sensu lato in ticks collected from migratory birds in Switzerland. *Applied and Environmental Microbiology*, Vol.72, No.1, (January 2006), pp. 976-979, ISSN 0099-2240

Ramamoorthi, N.; Narasimhan, S.; Pal, U.; Bao, F.; Yang, X.F.; Fish, D.; Anguita, J.; Norgard, M.V.; Kantor, F.S.; Anderson, J.F.; Koski, R.A. & Fikrig, E. (2005). The Lyme disease agent exploits a tick protein to infect the mammalian host. *Nature*, Vol.436, No.7050, (July 2005), pp. 573–577, ISSN 0028-0836

Randolph, S.E.; Gern, L. & Nuttall, P.A. Co-feeding ticks: Epidemiological significance for tick-borne pathogen transmission. *Parasitology today*, Vol.12, No.12, (December 1996), pp. 472-479, ISSN 0169-4758

Rauter, C. & Hartung, T. (2005). Prevalence of *Borrelia burgdorferi* sensu lato species in *Ixodes ricinus* ticks in Europe: a metaanalysis. *Applied and Environmental Microbiology*, Vol.71, No.11 (November 2005), pp. 7203–7216, ISSN 0099-2240Richter, D. & Matuschka, FR. (2006). Perpetuation of the Lyme disease spirochete *Borrelia lusitaniae* by lizards. *Applied and Environmental Microbiology*, Vol.72, No.7, (July 2006), pp. 4627–4632, ISSN 0099-2240

Richter, D.; Postic, D.; Sertour, N.; Livey, I.; Matuschka, F.-R. & Baranton, G. (2006). Delineation of *Borrelia burgdorferi* sensu lato species by multilocus sequence analysis and confirmation of the delineation of *Borrelia spielmanii* sp. nov. *International Journal of Systematic and Evolutionary Microbiology*, Vol.56, No.4, (April 2006), pp. 873–881, ISSN 1466-5026

Richter, D.; Schlee, D.B.; Allgöwer, R. & Matuschka, F.-R. (2004). Relationships of a novel Lyme disease spirochete, *Borrelia spielmanii* sp. nov., with its hosts in Central Europe. *Applied and Environmental Microbiology*, Vol.70, No.11, (November 2004), pp. 6414–6419, ISSN 0099-2240

Rosa, P. (2005). Lyme disease agent borrows a practical coat. *Nature Medicine*, Vol.11, Issue 8, (August 2005), pp. 831–832, ISSN 1078-8956

Rudenko, N.; Golovchenko, M.; Edwards, M. J. & Grubhoffer, L. (2005). Differential expression of *Ixodes ricinus* tick genes induced by blood feeding of *Borrelia burgdorferi* infection. *Journal of Medical Entomology*, Vol.42, No.1, (January 2005), pp. 36–41, ISSN 0022–2585

Rudenko, N.; Golovchenko, M.; Grubhoffer, L. & Oliver, H.J. (2009a). *Borrelia carolinensis* sp. nov., a new (14th) member of the *Borrelia burgdorferi* sensu lato complex from the south-eastern region of the United States. *Journal of Clinical Microbiology*, Vol.47, No.1, (January 2009), pp. 134–141, ISSN 0095-1137

Rudenko, N.; Golovchenko, M.; Lin, T.; Gao, L.; Grubhoffer, L. & Oliver, H.J. (2009b). Delineation of a new species of the *Borrelia burgdorferi* sensu lato complex, *Borrelia americana* sp. nov. *Journal of Clinical Microbiology*, Vol.47, No.12, (December 2009), pp. 3875–3880, ISSN 0095-1137

Rudenko, N.; Golovchenko, M.; Grubhoffer, L. & Oliver, J.H. (2011). Updates on *Borrelia burgdorferi* sensu lato complex with respect to public health. *Ticks and Tick-borne Diseases*, Vol.2, No.3, (September 2011), pp. 123–128, ISSN 1877-959X

Schwan T.G.; Schrumpf, M.E.; Karstens, R.H.; Clover, J.R.; Wong, J.; Daugherty, M.; Struthers, M. & Rosa P.A. (1993). Distribution and molecular analysis of Lyme disease spirochetes, *Borrelia burgdorferi*, isolated from ticks throughout California. *Journal of Clinical Microbiology*, Vol.31, No.12, (December 1993), pp. 3096-3108, ISSN 0095-1137

Smetanova, K.; Burri, C.; Perez, D.; Gern, L. & Kocianova, E. (2007). Detection and identification of *Borrelia burgdorferi* sensu lato genospecies in ticks from three different regions in Slovakia. *Wiener Klinische Wochenschrift*, Vol.119, No.17-18, (September 2007), pp. 534-537, ISSN 0043-5325

Sonenshine, D.E. (1991). *Biology of Ticks. Volume 1*, Oxford University Press, ISBN 0195059107, New York

Sood, S.K.; Salzman, M.B.; Johnson, B.J.; Happ, C.M.; Feig, K.; Carmody, L.; Rubin, L.G.; Hilton, E. & Piesman, J. (1997). Duration of tick attachment as a predictor of the risk of Lyme disease in an area in which Lyme disease is endemic. *Journal of Infectious Diseases*, Vol.175, No.4, (April 1997), pp. 996-999, ISSN 0022-1899

Špitalská, E.; Literák, I.; Sparagano, O.A.E.; Golovchenko, M. & Kocianová, E. (2006) Ticks (Ixodidae) from passerine birds in the Carpathian region. *Wiener Klinische Wochenschrift*, Vol.118, No.23-24, (December 2006), pp. 759-764, ISSN 0043-5325

Špitalská, E.; Literák, I.; Kocianová, E. & Taragel'ová, V. (2011).The Importance of *Ixodes arboricola* in Transmission of *Rickettsia* spp., *Anaplasma phagocytophilum*, and *Borrelia burgdorferi* sensu lato in the Czech Republic, Central Europe. *Vector-Borne and Zoonotic Diseases*, Vol.11, No.9, (September 2011), pp. 1235-1241, ISSN 1530-3667

Stefutkina, LF. (1989). Morphological and virological peculiarities of ixodid tick tissues and cells infection by the tick-borne encephalitis virus. *PhD-Thesis summary*, Moscow. 24 pp. (In Russian)

Stern, C.; Kaiser, A.; Maier, W.A. & Kampen, H. (2006). Die Rolle von Amsel (*Turdus merula*), Rotdrossel (*Turdus iliacus*) und Singdrossel (*Turdus philomelos*) als Blutwirte fur Zecken (Acari: Ixodidae) und Reservoirwirte fur vier Genospezies des *Borrelia burgdorferi*-Artenkomplexes. *Mitteilungen der Deutschen Gesellschaft für allgemeine und angewandte Entomologie*, Vol.15, (July 2006). pp. 349-356, ISSN 0344-9084

Taragelova, V.; Koci, J.; Hanincova, K.; Kurtenbach, K.; Derdakova, M.; Ogden, N.H.; Literak, I.; Kocianova, E. & Labuda, M. (2008). Blackbirds and song thrushes constitute a key reservoir of *Borrelia garinii*, the causative agent of borreliosis in Central Europe. *Applied and Environmental Microbiology*, Vol.74, No.4, (February 2008), pp. 1289-1293, ISSN 0099-2240

Vourc'h, G.; Boyard, C. & Barnouin, J. (2008). Mammal and bird species distribution at the woodland-pasture interface in relation to the circulation of ticks and pathogens. *Annals of the New York Academy of Sciences*, Vol.149, (December 2008), pp. 322-325, ISSN 1749-6632

Wagner-Jevseenko, O. (1958). Fortplanzung bei *Ornithodoros moubata* und genitale Ubertragung von *Borrelia duttoni*. *Acta Tropica*, Vol.15, No.2, (February 1958), pp. 118-168, ISSN 0001-706X

Wang, G.; van Dam, A.P.; Le Fleche, A.; Postic, D.; Péter, O.;Baranton, G.; de Boer, R.; Spanjaard, L. & Dankert, J. (1997). Genetic and phenotypic analysis of *Borrelia valaisiana* sp. nov. (*Borrelia* genomic groups VS116 and M19). *International Journal of Systematic Bacteriology*, Vol.47, No.4, (October 1997), pp. 926-932, ISSN 0020-7713

Wright, S.A.; Lemenager, D.A.; Tucker, J.R.; Armijos, M.V. & Yamamoto, S.A. (2006). An avian contribution to the presence of *Ixodes pacificus* (Acari: Ixodidae) and *Borrelia burgdorferi* on the Sutter Buttes of California. *Journal of Medical Entomology*, Vol.43, No.2, (March 2006), pp. 368-374, ISSN 0022-2585

Xu, G.; Fang, Q.Q.; Keirans, J.E. & Durden, L.A. (2003). Molecular phylogenetic analyses indicate that the *Ixodes ricinus* complex is a paraphyletic group. *Journal of Parasitology,* Vol.89, No.3, (June 2003), pp. 452–457, ISSN 0022-3395

Yeh, M.T.; Bak, J.M.; Hu, R.; Nicholson, M.C.; Kelly, C. & Mather, T.N. (1995). Determining the duration of *Ixodes scapularis* (Acari: Ixodidae) attachment to tick-bite victims. *Journal of Medical Entomology,* Vol.32, No.6, (November 1995), pp. 853–858, ISSN 0022-2585

Younsi, H.; Postic, D.; Baranton, G. & Bouattour, A. (2001). High prevalence of *Borrelia lusitaniae* in *Ixodes ricinus* ticks in Tunisia. *European Journal of Epidemiology,* Vol.7, No.1, (January 2001), pp. 53–56, ISSN 0393-2990

3

Advancement in *Borrelia burgdorferi* Antibody Testing: Comparative Immunoblot Assay (COMPASS)

András Lakos[1] and Erzsébet Igari[2]
[1]*Centre for Tick-borne Diseases, Outpatient Service and Laboratory*
[2]*Semmelweis University, Faculty of Medicine*
Hungary

1. Introduction

Since the discovery of the Borrelia burgdorferi s.l. (Bb) in 1982 (Burgdorfer et al., 1982), we can test antibodies against it. We could establish the diagnosis of Lyme borreliosis (Lb) and heal many-many patients by the help of this technique. Soon after the discovery of the pathogen, it became apparent that the serological tests are not sufficiently specific (Banyas, 1992; Cutler et al. 1994; Tuuminen et al., 2011). Generally, cross reacting antibodies (like in syphilitic patients) are accused for this type of bias (Craft et al., 1984; Raoult et al., 1989; Rath et al., 1994), but it is questionable whether most of the false positive reactions are originated from these cross reactive antibodies. The only diagnostic tool for supporting Lb in a routine laboratory is testing antibodies against Bb. Recently, the relatively cheap ELISA is most frequently used. This technique generally measures the amount of antibodies against different Bb antigens, and it is quantitative. Since ELISA detects more than one antibody we can not reveal which antibody gives the "positive" result. In an ELISA test the background noise and non specific reactions may be significant therefore it is generally accepted that test results provided by ELISA should be confirmed by Western (immuno) blot (Wb), this called as "two-step protocol" (CDC, 1995). Wb measures the different, most and less specific antibodies separately therefore it is considered to be more specific, but expensive method. The drawback of the Wb is that it is although qualitative but only semi quantitative. Most of the guidelines do not consider calculation with the band intensity at all (CDC, 1995; Dressler et al, 1993; Hauser et al, 1997). This mistake can be avoided by applying computer image analysis of Wb where intensity is also measured in comparison to factory given controls (Binnicker et al; 2008).

Problem 1/ In spite of that significant development is seen in methodology and test performance (Bacon et al., 2003; Porwancher et al., 2011; Steere et al., 2008), the test quality can be seriously different (Ang et al, 2011, Lakos, 1990; Marangoni et al., 2005; Nohlmans et al., 1994,). At least a part of the false positive results inevitably originate from a previous infection. The highest specificity ever published from an endemic population was 99.1%. (Goettner et al., 2005). Most of the tests have much lower specificity. Even the 99% specificity is excellent, we found that the positive predictive value (PPV) of this test is surprisingly low (less than 10%) when it is applied as a screening test in an average population living in endemic region (Lakos et al., 2010).

Since Bb antibody testing will result in at least 1% false positive result in endemic territories (practically in entire Europe), and basically, this false positivity is the consequence of a previous infection, this bias probably cannot be unravelled by newly developed serological techniques.

Problem 2/ The situation is even worth when Bb antibody testing is applied in people (forestry workers, hunters, orienteer, mushroom pickers and bee-keepers) with high risk for Lb. We found that among 1670 forestry workers 622 (37%) were seropositive and 280 (45%) of them was free of any symptoms and they also denied any symptom suggestive of Lb in their history. Therefore the PPV in this population is even lower, 1.8% (Lakos & Igari, 2011).

Problem 3/ Most of the guidelines follow the case definition of EM published by CDC (CDC, 2008) and EUCALB (Stanek et al., 1996). But there is no instruction what a clinician should do in a case when the rash does not fulfil the diagnostic criteria of EM but otherwise Bb infection can not be ruled out safely. In such cases, clinicians order antibiotic treatment for sure what is sure. Delusion is very probable in such cases and the consequences are regularly serious (Steere et al., 2004). How can we prove that the patient does not need antibiotic treatment?

Problem 4/ It is a basic rule that a symptom free patient must not be treated with antibiotics just because of a "positive" serological result. A competent physician neither treats a symptom free patient with a previous symptom suggestive of Lb. How can one sure that being free of symptoms means being free of infection?

Problem 5/ Facial palsy is a frequent complication of Lb. Tick bite usually resides behind the ear in these cases, therefore rarely recognised. EM is usually missing, therefore the only diagnostic tool is Bb antibody testing. Since facial palsy is an early complication, the antibody reaction is still negative in many cases. Situation is complicated by steroid treatment what is usually applied based on studies showing facial palsy improved by corticosteroids (Numthavaj et al., 2011; Sullivan et al., 2007). This treatment may modify antibody reaction and help propagation of Bb. The Lyme spirochete frequently invades the central nervous system but in spite of that it does not result in apparent clinical symptoms (Ackermann et al., 1984; Pachner & Steere, 1984). Facial palsy caused by Bb infection is usually benign, self limited illness. These increase the chance of being hidden the origin of the disease. What should a doctor do when the serology is negative shortly after the debut of facial palsy?

Problem 6/ Studies have been published supporting that Bb is able to survive the adequate antibiotic treatment (Kannian et al., 2007; Maraspin et al., 2002; Steere & Angelis, 2006; Wormser et al., 2003). To prove this in a given patient, biopsies and culture or PCR should be applied but sensitivity of these techniques after treatment is questionable. These methods are expensive, usually invasive and time consuming; therefore they are inappropriate for routine diagnostics. What about serology? Is it the right way for demonstration of Bb survival?

Problem 7/ It is generally accepted that demonstration of intrathecal antibody production is necessary for supporting neuroborreliosis. The basic problem is that leakage of the blood-brain barrier may result in appearance of the peripherally produced immunoglobulin in the cerebrospinal fluid (CSF). We should differentiate between the intrathecally and peripherally produced antibodies presented in the CSF. Some techniques have been developed for solve this problem. Most of these apply four measurements (e.g. serum IgG anti-Bb antibodies / total serum IgG antibodies and CSF IgG anti-Bb antibodies / total CSF IgG antibodies).

Mathematical equations were developed as well as arbitrarily defined factors were applied and the usefulness of these was supported by empirical data (Halperin et al., 1991; Kaiser, 2000; Wilske et al., 1986). The more measurements we take, the more mistakes we can make. The most serious mistakes may present in cases where the amounts of immunoglobulins are excessively low or high as just this situation is typical for Bb infected patient without neuroborreliosis and the non-Lyme patients. What possibilities we have to achieve safer results with fewer measurements?

Problem 8/ A lot of papers show that about 10% of the adequately treated patients develop subjective symptoms (fatigue, cognitive impairment and musculoskeletal pain) months or years later. These complaints named "post Lyme syndrome" can not be improved by antibiotic treatments (Klempner et al., 2001, Marques, 2008; Wormser et al, 2006). But we can not rule out that these symptoms are resulted from surviving Bb. Ineffectiveness of antibiotic treatment(s) is not enough for proving that post Lyme syndrome is not a consequence of long lasting Bb infection. Could we find more support to clarify this?

Problem 9/ A lot of papers on the effectiveness of antibiotic treatment in Lb have been published but exaggerated guidelines appeared. For example, 10 days (Wormser et al., 2003) versus 30 days (Stanek & Strle, 2003) doxycyclin treatment were also suggested. Moreover we found a study applying 11 months long treatment (Donta, 1997). In contrast, azithromycin described to be effective in a five day course (Arnez et al., 2002, Hunfeld et al., 2005). The situation is more complicated since the treatments are suggested to be shorter in the early forms than in the later. What is the reason of the difference? Is there any evidence for this practice? More recently, neuroborreliosis is suggested to be treated by doxycycline with a similar dose as we use it in the treatment of EM. With this treatment we may not achieve MIC or MBC levels of some Bb isolations in the CSF (Baradaran-Dilmaghani & Stanek, 1996; Karlsson et al., 1996; Kleibeuker et al., 2009). Treatment of pregnant women is also a special issue. The guideline of IDSA (Infectious Disease Society of America) claims that pregnant women should be treated by the same dose of amoxicillin as other Lyme patients (3x500mg/die) (Wormser et al., 2006). In turn of this statement the metabolism of amoxicillin is faster in pregnancy, moreover the increased body weight and relatively higher amount of body fluid result in lower antibiotic level than needed (Andrew et al., 2007). We found that orally treated pregnant women has almost the same chance for adverse outcome as the untreated women in contrast with the treatment with ceftriaxone, that resulted in almost 100% safe in preventing the complications (Lakos & Solymosi, 2010). Lb is usually benign and self limited disease, therefore judgement of the effectiveness of an antibiotic treatment would need a study on a rather big population. Clinical improvement does not imply per se that microbiological cure was also achieved. On the contrary, if the patient complains for persistent or relapsed symptoms it does not necessarily mean that Bb survived the antibiotic treatment. Designing of a double blind study for the comparative effectiveness of an antibiotic treatment is quite complicated. Since the photosensitive reaction of doxycycline we easily recognise which treatment was applied before the patient would sound. The nasal redness is very characteristic sign of doxycycline treatment during the summer (i.e. Lyme) season and rarely missing. The double blind setting is definitely hurt when ceftriaxone treatment is tested since the characteristic smell of the antibiotic discloses the real drug for the patient and physician as well. Therefore a laboratory method would be better to test the effectiveness of the antibiotic instead of analysis of the subjective data of symptoms.

We developed the comparative immunoblot assay (COMPASS) to solve the above problems.

2. Methods

2.1 Western (immuno) blot

Bb (strain ACA1) was disintegrated by ultrasound than proteins were separated by SDS polyacrylamide gel ELFO. These proteins were transferred (blotted) to a polyvinyl difluorid membrane. This membrane is more durable than the gel, and the immunological reaction is performed on this membrane, that is the first layer. We put on the diluted serum or CSF sample to be tested. The antibodies strongly connected to the antigens therefore the repeated washing can eliminate all the serum components except the bound antibodies. The next step is the application of an anti-human immunoglobulin which was produced by an animal. This was conjugated by the producer factory with an enzyme which can develop the colouring reagent that is insoluble and remains in the membrane, showing the location of the bound antibodies (bands) as well the intensity of the binding. This intensity reflects to the concentration of bound antibodies. We waited for the development of the appropriate intensity than we apply the stop reagent, the last step of the serological reaction. The band intensity is merely influenced by the quality and concentrations of each layer. We establish the optimal concentration of each layer by checker board dilution. The location of a given antigen/antibody was originally defined with the help of monoclonal antibodies. Than we selected positive control samples for IgG and IgM and signed the appropriate molecular weights to a scanned image of these positive control samples. With the help of this scanned and signed image we can easily locate the bands during the routine examinations. We subjectively judge the intensity of the bands comparing the control samples. The positivity/negativity (i.e. cut-off) of a given Wb test can be defined by different ways. We tested 300 clinically defined Lyme patients (EM, lymphocytic meningoradiculitis and acrodermatitis chronica atrophicans - ACA) and 300 controls (healthy blood donors, infants and patients with autoimmune diseases). Based on these studies, the most specific bands were: 23, 29, 35, 44, 47, 49, 93 kDa molecular weights in IgG; 23 and 41 kDa in IgM. We analysed also the intensity of the bands (Lakos & Granström, 1997).

2.2 COMPASS

This method was described earlier in some respect. Accordingly, in most cases, two samples were drawn with an interval. The first sample was stored in a deep freezer and then tested together with the second sample when it was drawn later. These samples are tested side by side in Wb, therefore the difference or sameness can safely be judged, and the technical bias is practically avoided. These are partly described in previous papers (Lakos et al., 1997, 2005, 2008). We evaluate the difference between the samples and not the "positivity/negativity". Progression means persistent, lack of progression represents past infection. There are specific applications of COMPASS when the two samples drawn on the same day i.e. testing intrathecal antibody production, when serum and CSF samples are compared or testing intrauterine infection when serum samples of the mother and the newborn are compared. Sample pairs are always tested side by side.

2.3 Patients

There were some patients who remained untreated; their data are extremely useful for improving our knowledge on that how Bb antibodies develop in time. Patients remained untreated from different reasons: some of them refused the antibiotic treatment and used alternative medicine, e.g. homeopathy. In some other, the first sign of EM was not typical or smaller than 5cm in diameter but later the clinical appearance turned to be definitive. There were patients who had no symptoms at the first visit but because of multiple tick bite we tested a serum sample with negative result. Weeks later EM developed and the second sample was drawn.

2.4 Ethics

This study was approved by the Scientific and Ethical Committee of Medical Research Council (2409-0/2011-EKU - 66PI/11), based on the review of the detailed description (objective, background, hypothesis, study design - collecting patients, their clinical and laboratory data, the number and age of the participant patients). All patients provided a written informed consent: "I give my permission to Dr. Lakos to use the clinical and laboratory data collected on my (or my child's) illness for scientific analysis without mentioning my name and other personal information. This personal information must not be shared with other person. I am aware that have the right to withdraw my permission before the study will be closed." The study complied with the principles laid down in the Declaration of Helsinki.

3. Examples

In this section we illustrate the usefulness of COMPASS in different situations, and present some cases to show the process of antibody response to Bb infection in untreated patients.

3.1 COMPASS for serological confirmation of microbiological cure

3.1.1 Example 1

A, 26.09.1996. The 80 years old woman showed typical clinical signs of ACA. The first serum sample was drawn 18 months after the first treatment administered at another institute. She received IV penicillin for 8 days than 1x100mg doxycycline orally for 7 days. The size of the inflamed region decreased but the pain remained at the region of ACA. Concerning the extreme positive antibody response and complains we prescribed doxycycline and azithromycin. A year later arthralgia and polyneuropathy developed; therefore we ordered antibiotic treatments again.

B, 24.02.2000. By this time she received 5 courses of antibiotics altogether for 137 days, among these ceftriaxone was administered in twice regimens.

C, 21.05.2002. This is the last sample, almost 6 years after the first. COMPASS shows the definitive serological regression in spite of that the last sample is still strongly positive. Most of the bands faded, antibody against OspC disappeared (arrows).

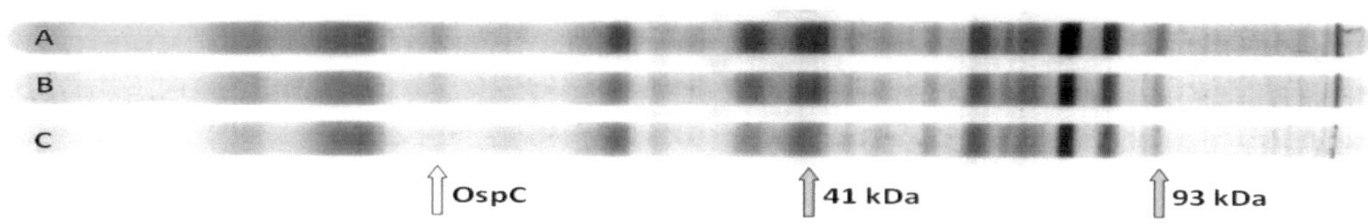

Fig. 1. Serological follow up in a patient with ACA (IgG)

3.1.2 Example 2

A, 23.08.2010. Patient was treated with amoxicillin for EM.

B, 18.06.2011. The intensity remained unchanged in all but one bands. In spite of the result is still positive, microbiological cure is proven.

Fig. 2. Clinical and serological recovery (IgG)

3.1.3 Example 3

A, 16.08.2010. EM located behind the knee and accompanied by serious pain in the leg. He was treated with doxycycline for 40 days 100mg b.i.d.

B, 18.06.2011. He is free of any symptoms. Although the result is still positive but there is no progression, and the antibody against the 44kDa protein decreased, therefore microbiological cure is proven.

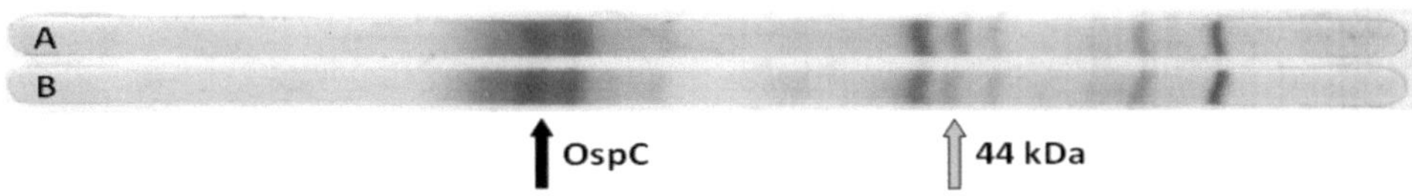

Fig. 3. Another example for clinical and serological recovery (IgG)

3.1.4 Example 4

She had a typical EM from May to October 2009, and visited our Centre shortly after the abortion of her 8 weeks old pregnancy. The EM was still high coloured, and disappeared during amoxicillin treatment.

A, 22.07.2010. This sample was drawn nine months after the treatment for proving microbiological cure.

B, 02.02.2011. She asked for serology because of arthralgia. Since no definitive progression was seen, she was not retreated.

C, 15.06.2011. The woman asked for this test before planning a new pregnancy. A definitive decrease is seen in the reaction against the 14kDa protein. The minimal progression in the 41kDa (flagellar) antibody turned to be temporary. This is a good example for that serological regression may be seen long after the treatment.

Fig. 4. Another example for clinical and serological recovery (IgG)

3.1.5 Example 5

Tetraplegia developed gradually with chronic lymphocytic meningitis in April 1994.

He was treated with ceftriaxone in February 1995, than with doxycycline in November 1997. He improved a lot, able to walk without any support but clumsiness in coordination progressed since a year.

A, 01.12.1997.

B, 21.03.2005.

C, 09.06.2011. This is a good example for that many years after healing of a serious, long lasting Bb infection the serological result is still strongly positive. Proving the microbiological cure would not be possible without COMPASS which shows moderate decrease in antibody response.

Fig. 5. Healing of progressive Borrelia encephalomyelitis (IgG)

3.2 COMPASS suggesting Borrelia survival

3.2.1 Example 1

A, 11.08.2010. EM started 25 days before sampling. The IgM serology was strongly positive. She was treated with amoxicillin 1000mg t.i.d.

B, 08.12.2010. The next sample showed serological progression but she was not retreated.

C, 15.06.2011. In the third sample a minimal further progression is shown (striped arrow). Another antibiotic treatment was prescribed.

Fig. 6. Serological progression after clinically successful treatment of EM (IgG)

3.2.2 Example 2

Arthritis of the right knee developed in April, 2010. Other large joints became intermittently swollen.

A, 05.04.2011. He was treated with 100mg doxycycline b.i.d., but the arthritis persisted. Ceftriaxone was ordered 1x2g IV for 15 days. The inflammation seemed to be healed but one week after finishing the treatment left knee became swollen again (17.06.2011.).

B, 23.06.2011. Almost every band shows progression (striped arrows) but some new bands also appeared (dotted arrows). We have not seen similar serological progression after successful treatment.

This example also represents that the very strong reaction can progress to a more reactive form. Lyme arthritis always accompanied by similarly strong antibody reaction as in acrodermatitis chronica atrophicans and progressive encephalomyelitis.

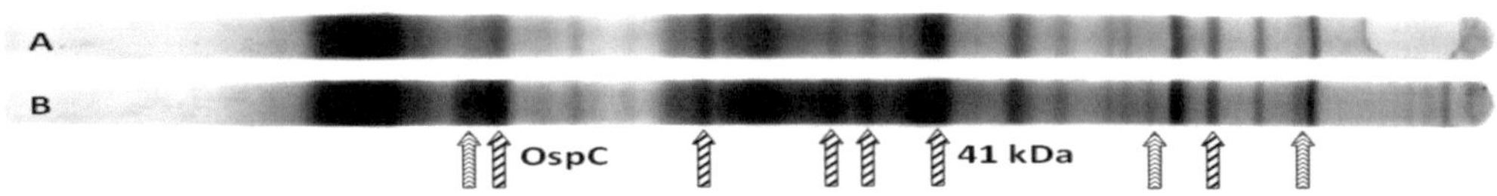

Fig. 7. Seroprogression after the ineffective treatment of Lyme arthritis (IgG)

3.2.3 Example 3

A, 09.08.2010. EM started 4 days before sampling. He was treated with amoxicillin for 20 days.

B, 02.12.2010. Minimal progression was seen in OspC (striped arrow), but he was not retreated at this time.

C, 22.06.2011. Further progression is seen in 44kDa antibody. Treatment was ordered.

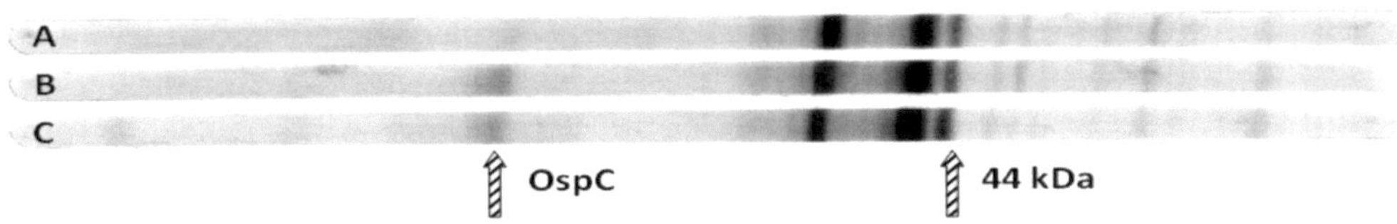

Fig. 8. Seroprogression after clinically successful treatment (IgG)

3.2.4 Example 4

A, 30.09.2010. A tick was recognised behind the ear one month before. Peripheral facial palsy started three days before sampling. Strong reaction was seen in IgM. Facial palsy was healed one week after starting the ceftriaxone therapy (2g IV, per day).

B, 09.12.2010. Definitive progression was seen in IgG but antibiotic treatment was not ordered at this time.

C, 15.06.2011. Further progression is seen, antibiotic treatment was prescribed.

Fig. 9. Serological progression after clinically successful treatment (IgG)

3.2.5 Example 5

A, 30.08.2010. She was treated with two courses (17 days in total) of azithromycin because of peripheral facial palsy with strong positive Bb antibody IgM reaction. She visited our Centre one week after healing of the palsy and just after finishing the treatment.

B, 30.11.2010. Serological regression was visible in the 44kDa band.

C, 31.05.2011. Progression appeared (arrow) half year later in the same band. We assessed this phenomenon - ie. the transitory serological regression followed by progression - as a sign of Bb survival. The patient was retreated.

Fig. 10. Clinically successful treatment of facial palsy with serological progression (IgG)

3.2.6 Example 6

EM started on 07.06.2011., one day after the tick bite.

A, 23.06.2011. She visited our Centre with an EM 5cm in diameter and refused antibiotics since homeopathic treatment was thought to be safer.

B, 21.07.2011. The EM increased to 60cm. Faint serological progression was seen only in IgM. According to our in-house standards this result was only borderline.

Fig. 11. EM treated with homeopathy (IgM)

3.2.7 Example 7

EM started in September, 2010 disappeared without any treatment by the end of February, 2011.

A, 28.03.2011. Immunoblot showed very strong antibody reaction.

B, 04.08.2011. COMPASS suggested the survival of Bb in spite of that the patient remained free of symptom. Almost every band became more intense and some new bands appeared.

C, Positive control sample is also included for comparison of the band intensity.

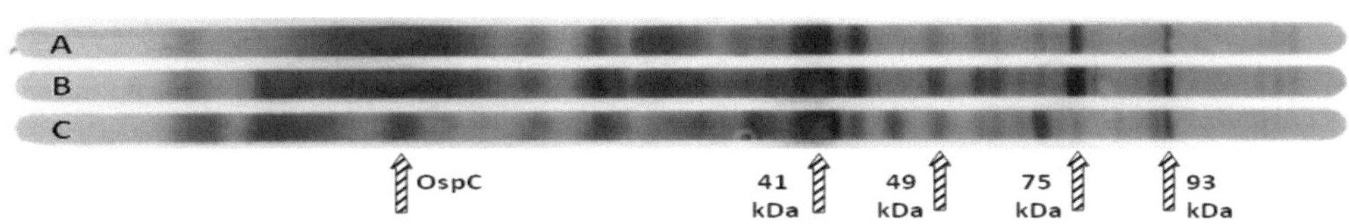

Fig. 12. Untreated erythema migrans (IgG)

3.3 COMPASS in possible relapse of Lyme borreliosis

3.3.1 Example 1

A, 06.07.2008. The patient visited our Centre with EM.

B, 14.06.2011. COMPASS showed serological regression in OspC while the other bands remained unchanged four months after the debut of arthralgia. Our decision was that the new complains are not related to the previous Bb infection.

Fig. 13. No relapse (IgG)

3.3.2 Example 2

Between November 2009 and September 2010 this patient was treated with five courses of antibiotics in other institutes since he was found to be seropositive and had complains of paraesthesia, fatigue and abnormal cardiac palpitation. There was a probable EM in her history in around 1996.

A, 09.09.2010. There are several faint bands in this lane, suggesting the positive reaction is a result of immune memory but not an active Bb infection.

B, 12.05.2011. Eight months later the result is still „positive" but serological regression is visible in the 37kDa band. Actual Bb infection was ruled out.

Fig. 14. No actual Lb in spite of the "positive" serological reaction (IgG)

3.4 COMPASS for screening in pregnancy after tick bite

3.4.1 Example 1

A, 08.06.2011. This sample was drawn at the 39th week of pregnancy, 17 days after a tick bite.

B, 27.06.2011. An erythema started and developed to a typical EM five days after the previous sampling. Minimal seroprogression is visible (striped arrows).

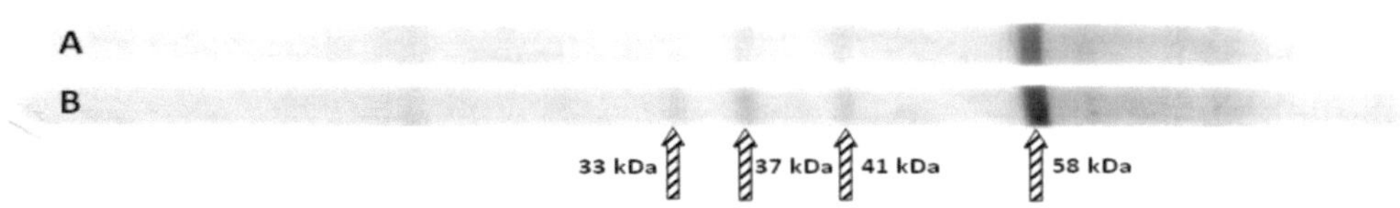

Fig. 15. Seroprogression with interval of 19 days (IgM)

3.4.2 Example 2

A, 23.06.2011. Sample of this patient with 14 weeks of pregnancy was drawn 17 days after a tick bite. There was no antibody response at this time.

B, 21.07.2011. Antibody response progressed definitively 28 days later. She was treated with ceftriaxone in spite of being free of symptoms.

Fig. 16. Serological progression after a tick bite in pregnancy (IgG)

Fig. 17. Minimal amount of serological progression in IgM (same patient)

3.5 COMPASS for screening - after multiple tick bites

3.5.1 Example 1

A, 01.06.2011. This test was done after ten tick bites (30.05.2011.). We observed a borderline reaction.

B, 15.06.2011. This sample was drawn when an EM developed to 11cm in diameter.

Fig. 18. Seroprogression after 14 days (IgM)

3.6 COMPASS in atypical erythema migrans

3.6.1 Example 1

A, 15.06.2011. Rapidly progressing, significantly swollen, painful erythema shaped to 4cm after a probable tick bite (27.05.2011.). Typical EM 7cm in diameter developed eight days later.

B, 23.06.2011. The second sample is still negative but the serological progression is definitive.

Fig. 19. Seroprogression within 8 days (IgM)

3.7 COMPASS in facial palsy

3.7.1 Example 1

A, 17.01.2011. Facial palsy started in November 2010. The patient was treated with methylprednisolone and healed in four days. The result was in the negative range.

B, 23.03.2011. He came back two months later. Serological progression in the 21kDa band suggests active Bb infection, antibiotic treatment was started. This is a good example for that one band may decrease while another increase in intensity. That is why ELISA is not an appropriate method for comparative assay since the regression in a particular band may be compensated by the progression of another band.

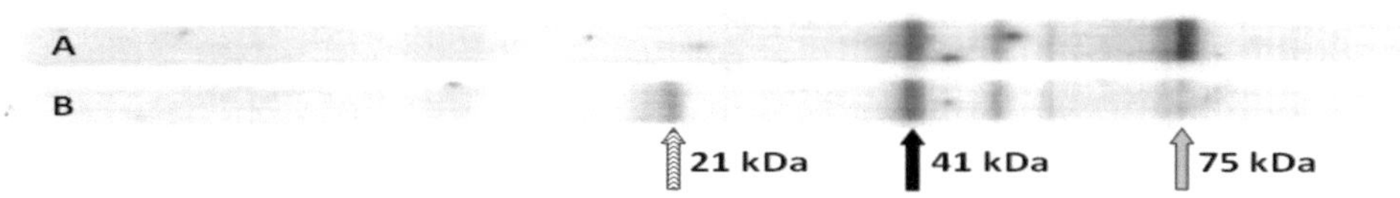

Fig. 20. Seroprogression in a symptom free patient after peripheral facial palsy (IgG)

3.8 COMPASS for evaluating intrathecal *Borrelia burgdorferi* s.l. antibody production

3.8.1 Example 1

There is a consensus regarding the demonstration of intrathecal antibody production as the currently most reliable diagnostic tool for Lyme disease with neurological involvement. Based on our study, intrathecal antibody production was considered to be positive if the immunoblot pattern observed clearly differed between the serum and the CSF sample in a pair. The difference could consist of bands present in CSF but not in serum or, conversely, bands that were present in serum were lacking in CSF, while at least one of the corresponding bands in the CSF was equally or more intense than in the serum. In addition to these differences, the intensity of the bands were also used as diagnostic criterion, if the difference was so disproportionate that a theoretical dilution or concentration of either the samples could not result in the same pattern as the other sample of the pair (Lakos et al, 2005).

In this example, there is a band (39kDa) in the CSF (C) missing from the serum (S) while an inverse situation is seen in the 24kDa band.

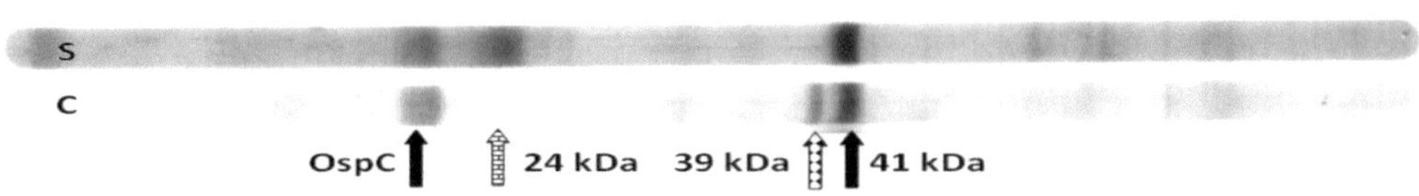

Fig. 21. Neuroborreliosis (lymphocytic meningoradiculits, Bannwarth's syndrome - IgM)

In IgG, there is a strong difference between serum and CSF in the 41 and the 93kDa bands, while the intensity of 47kDa almost the same in the serum and in the CSF. In this case both IgM and IgG represent the intrathecal Bb antibody synthesis, but either of them would fulfil the diagnostic criterion of proving the neuroborreliosis.

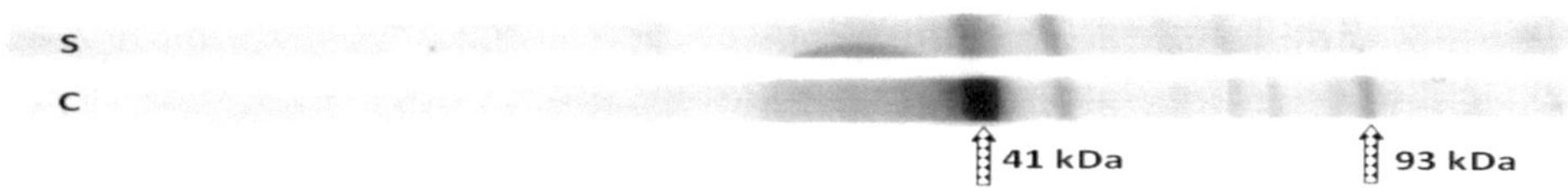

Fig. 22. Same patient (IgG)

3.8.2 Example 2

19.12.2010. Epilepsy developed in this forestry worker, and positive Bb antibody IgG reaction was found in the serum and CSF in another institute. In the CSF, only very faint bands are found, and they mirror the band pattern of the serum. There is no intrathecal antibody production, therefore neuroborreliosis is ruled out. For comparison, the positive control sample is included to illustrate that the bands of the forestry worker, although there are many, they are faint and dim. This is typical late sign for the previously healed long lasting or repeated Bb infection as it frequently seen in high risk patients.

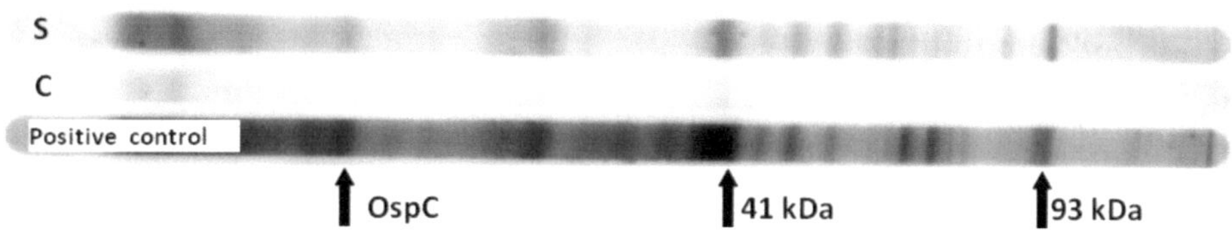

Fig. 23. Serum and CSF pair of a forestry worker (IgG). Neuroborreliosis is excluded.

3.8.3 Example 3

A, 28.11.2010. This forestry worker was tested because of isolated hypoglossal palsy started a year before the first sampling. Even there are definitive bands in the CSF (C) (an ELISA test was IgG positive in another institute), they wanly mirror the band pattern of the serum (S), therefore there is no sign of intrathecal Bb antibody synthesis, and we ruled out neuroborreliosis. He did not get antibiotic treatment.

B, 22.07.2011. The repeated COMPASS shows no change, supporting that our previous opinion was correct. The "positive" ELISA reaction originated from leakage of the blood-brain barrier.

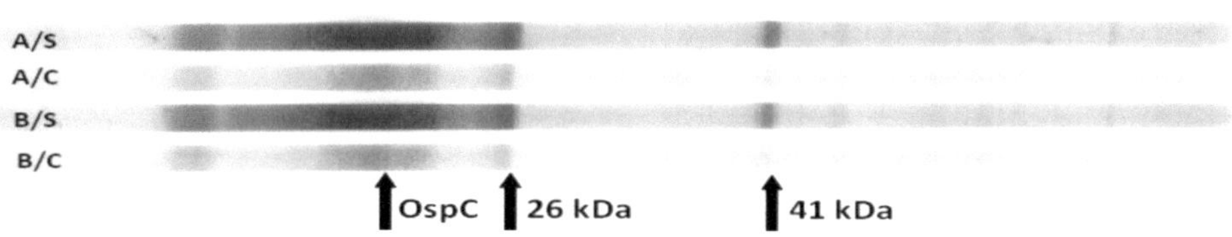

Fig. 24. Serum and cerebrospinal fluid pair of a forestry worker with positive reaction in both samples but without neuroborreliosis (IgG)

3.9 COMPASS in high risk patients

3.9.1 Example 1

A, 25.06.1992. He was first tested as a member of a survey among forestry workers. He was free of any symptoms at that time. The characteristic of WB (dim bands) and COMPASS applied with an interval of six months (not shown) suggested that Bb infection healed earlier.

B, 07.04.1999. Arthralgia started in 1999 but based on COMPASS, we ruled out the possibility of a present infection. In contrast, his samples were regularly tested as positive in other labs, and he was regularly treated with antibiotics. He received doxycycline and ceftriaxone courses ten times during the following 2 years.

C, 21.05.2002. In May 2002 his complains seriously worsened. Based on COMPASS, we definitely ruled out an active Borrelia infection but antibiotic treatments were still repeatedly prescribed by other physicians.

In March, 2003 osteosarcoma was disclosed and the patient died in September 2003.

Fig. 25. Serological follow up in a forestry worker with previously healed Bb infection died of osteosarcoma recognized too late (IgG)

3.9.2 Example 2

A, 07.07.2010. This symptom free forestry worker was screened and found to be positive in other institute. He was not treated with antibiotic. The dim bands suggested previous and long lasting but already healed infection. We repeated the test.

B, 16.05.2011. The unchanged band pattern of the second sample proved our original opinion: there is no actual Bb infection.

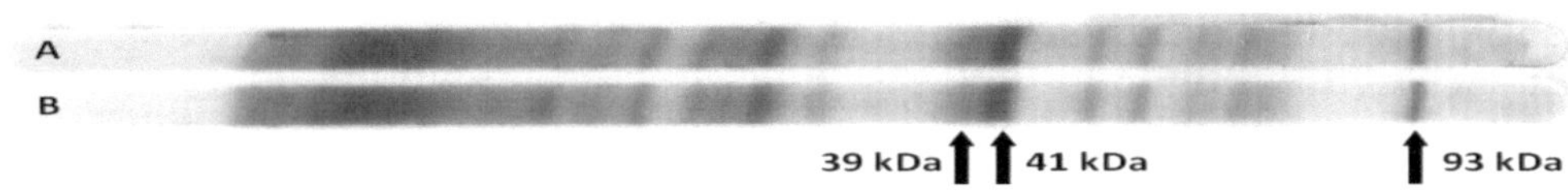

Fig. 26. No actual Bb infection in spite of the positive serological result (IgG)

3.10 COMPASS in reinfection

3.10.1 Example 1

A, 16.07.2008. This sample was drawn one month after 10 tick bites, but the result was negative at this time.

B, 29.06.2011. Almost three years later, the second sample was drawn 9 days after 40 spots of typical EM appeared as a result of new tick-bites. This example represent that multiple EM always present with extremely positive IgM reaction and this is shown at the very early stage of the clinical symptom.

Fig. 27. Intensive seroprogression in IgM following a multiple EM

3.10.2 Example 2

A, 20.10.2010. Parkinson's syndrome was started after an EM, two years before the first sampling. Based on the result, even positive, but faint and dim bands, chronic neuroborreliosis was ruled out.

B, 23.06.2011. The second sample was drawn on the day of recognition of a new EM with 6cm in diameter, 10 days after a tick bite. The serological progression was evident.

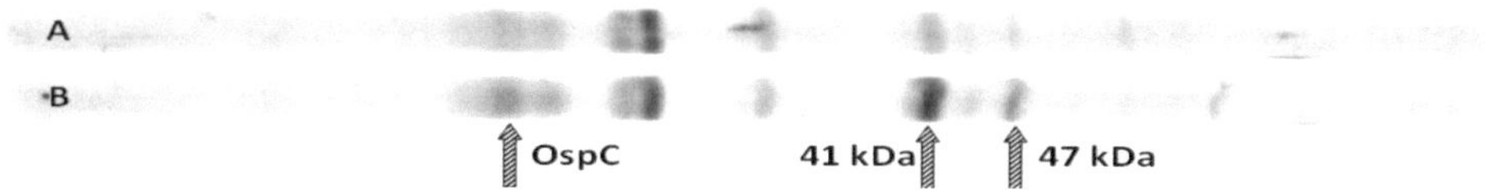

Fig. 28. Serological progression after reinfection (IgG)

3.10.3 Example 3

In this hunter, EM was started in September 2005. Healed, but 18 months later arthralgia developed.

A, 18.07.2007. The band pattern (dim and faint bands) was typical for already healed, previous Bb infection. Actual Lb was ruled out.

B, 15.06.2011. A giant EM, 100cm in diameter recognised one week ago. The band pattern is typical for reinfection: some of the previous bands disappeared but new bands presented. In the second sample, the bands are more intensive than they were in the previous sample.

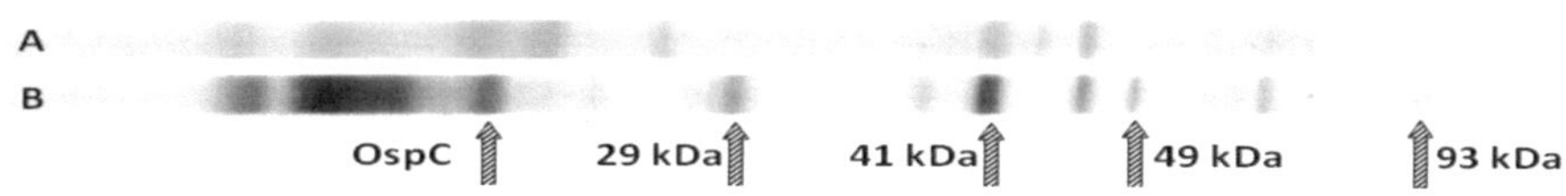

Fig. 29. Reinfection in a hunter (IgG)

3.10.4 Example 4

A, 31.08.2010. This patient was followed because of an earlier EM (May, 2010).

B, 04.04.2011. Three weeks before this sampling an itchy erythema developed with 15cm in diameter, tick bite was not recognised. The spot fainted a week ago. The serological progression in IgM proved that the patient has actual Bb infection and antibiotic was prescribed.

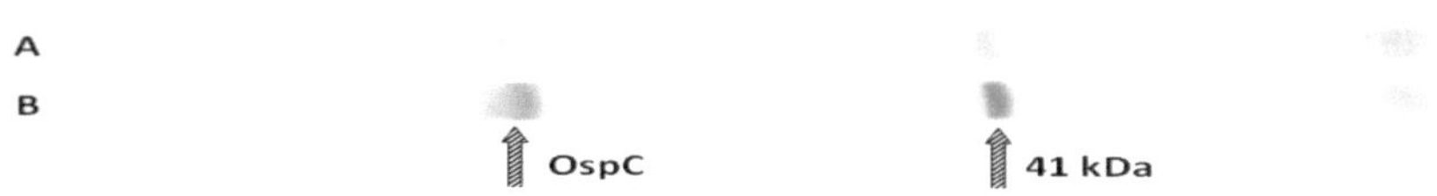

Fig. 30. Signs of reinfection (IgM)

3.11 COMPASS in probable false positive serological reaction

3.11.1 Example 1

This patient was examined because she had positive IgM Borrelia immunoblot results in other lab.

A, 23.05.2011. Our test also showed positive reaction in IgM but her symptom (eczema) did not suggest Lb. Therefore, we did not treat her with antibiotic in spite of the positive serological result.

B, 28.06.2011. Instead, we repeated the test. The COMPASS did not reveal progression in IgG neither changes in IgM. This suggests that the patient had false positive antibody reaction and actual Bb infection was ruled out.

Fig. 31. Patient with false positive IgM reaction with no change in COMPASS

3.12 COMPASS for testing possible foetal Borrelia infection

3.12.1 Example 1

A, 23.06.2010. This patient is a pregnant woman with EM, in the end of first trimester. We treated her with ceftriaxone.

B, 24.01.2011. This sample was collected at the day of delivery.

C, 24.01.2011. Cord blood sample of the newborn. Minimal amount of serological regression is seen after 7 months. The band pattern of the newborn is exactly mirrors the band pattern of the mother. IgM was completely negative. Our opinion was that the foetus did not acquire Bb infection.

Fig. 32. COMPASS in maternal and newborn samples (IgG)

3.12.2 Example 2

Mother recognised her EM at her 32nd week of pregnancy. She was treated with ceftriaxone only for 11 days because of allergic reaction.

A, 29.06.2011. The mother still had a strong reaction in 41kDa IgM at the time of delivery.

B, 29.06.2011. But the newborn had no antibody in IgM (neither in IgG), representing that he did not get the infection. Note: IgM can not cross the placental barrier, therefore IgM antibodies in the newborn sample would mean foetal infection - but this was not the case.

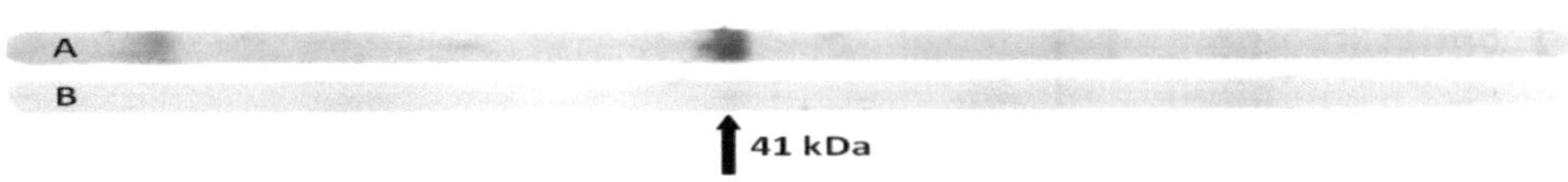

Fig. 33. After healing of the maternal EM, mother still has strong band in IgM, but the newborn has no antibody as a sign of that he has not been infected.

3.12.3 Example 3

This patient recognised an EM at the time of her twenty-fourth week of pregnancy.

A, 18.11.2009. This is a sample drawn three months after the treatment.

B, 15.12.2009. Cord blood sample. Even the newborn is also positive in IgG, all bands mirror the band pattern of the mother. The foetus has not been infected.

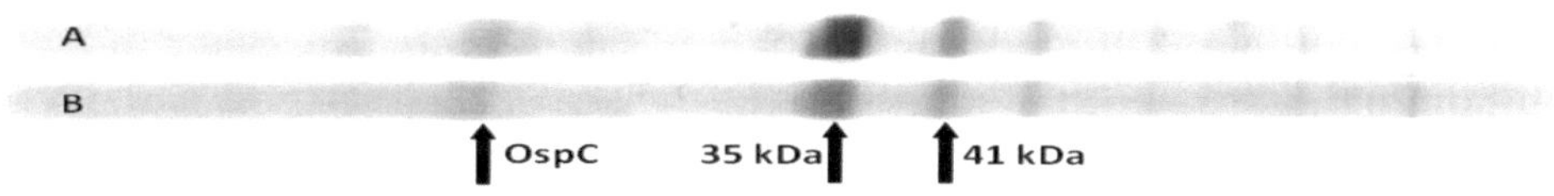

Fig. 34. Maternal and newborn samples (IgG)

4. Discussion

Here we presented a method which is useful for any laboratory working with WB, without any investment. We believe that this method significantly improve the serological diagnosis of Lb and can solve most of the problems may occur in this field. The method is basically simple, comparison of two samples tested side by side by WB. Testing two samples drawn with an interval we can prove the microbiological cure and this results in satisfaction of the patients and prevents abuse of antibiotics and repeated testing. Also we can find those patients who have persistent infection, after a retreatment their microbiological cure can be proven at the end.

Uncountable studies have published on serological diagnosis of Lb and many of them dealt with serological regression after treatment. We are not aware of a single paper on the description of the serological progression detected by Wb in treated or untreated Bb infected patients. We found only one similar study where Toxoplasma gondii WB of immunocompromised patients were studied in a similar setting as our COMPASS (Ashburn et al., 1998). Another work on untreated and spontaneously healed Lb patients was published but only the serological regression was detected by ELISA (Szer et al., 1991).

Since the discovery of Lb we are aware of that the infection may be generalized and became chronic, therefore the diagnosis of the disease is equal to the introduction of antibiotic treatment. This treatment aborts the antibody response. Therefore it is a rare occasion when we can observe the serological progression, the development of the antibody response in the course of time. This observation may improve in finding specific antigens. In contrast to the USA we have no consensus on which antibodies are the best for supporting the diagnosis of Lb in Europe (Robertson et al., 2000). It is obvious that the observation of the characteristics of serological progression could help to find the best antibodies for diagnostic purposes. If we can find antibodies progressing in the untreated patients in contrast to the controls, these should be considered specific. Our examples show that some specific antibodies decrease during the serological progression. We think this phenomenon is not generally known. Detecting the progressing antibodies in untreated patients may indicate of specificity irrespectively of that the result is otherwise "positive" or "negative". It should be stressed that the negative serological result does not rule out the possibility of Lb during the first two months of the infection, as positive result does not necessarily imply actual Bb infection since this can also reflect to a previous - many times asymptomatic - infection.

Consequently, testing only one sample is not enough for definitive diagnosis in many if not most case. In contrast, testing of a sample pair, the serological progression strongly supports the actual infection and the unchanged reaction represents the opposite. Ideally, a study on a regularly tested, untreated group of patients with clinically characteristic sign of Lb could answer that what the optimal interval is for drawing the sample pairs and which and how intensive antibodies appear during time. Since this is ethically nonsense, only the regular collection of these data on clinical and laboratory praxis can help.

Here we presented untreated patients where the amount of the antibodies and/or the number of the bands increased with time. It is clear that the serodiagnosis is more accurate when we compare the actual antibody response with a previous sample than with the cut-off. We presume that the serological progression proves the active, present infection (except some well defined situation, such as shortly after the antibiotic treatment). When the antibody profile is in the positive range but remains unchanged it means that the antibodies originate from a previous, already healed infection. COMPASS may increase the specificity of Bb antibody testing since it can discriminate past, healed and present, active infection. Confusion of these two possibilities of the positive reaction results in low PPV of serological tests. Application of COMPASS can avoid the problem of that different tests set up the cut-off levels in different ways.

The main topic of this study is to help physicians and microbiologists in those cases where the clinical picture is suggestive for Lb but ambiguous. It is generally accepted that clinical case definition of EM consists of at least 5cm in diameter, gradually enlarging rash. Morphea, tinea, Schamberg purpura, granuloma anulare, erythema nodosum, and allergic reaction to the tick itself may fulfil these criteria in particular cases. Not every clinician is sufficiently experienced to be able to distinguish these symptoms from EM and also, there are situations where competent clinicians also have to face diagnostic problems. Serology is the only tool for supporting the diagnosis in doubtful cases. Antibody response is regularly missing in the early cases. A few weeks later the progression in the antibody reaction can prove the Bb infection right before the serological result became "positive".

We have to face confusion not only in cases with early symptoms suspect to Lb where neither clinical signs nor serology can help. An old forestry worker probably has strong antibody reaction to Bb and also complains of musculoskeletal symptom. Is there a causal relation? COMPASS can solve the problem: if the serological progression is missing in the untreated worker, Bb infection can be ruled out.

Every guideline emphasizes that Lb should be based on characteristic clinical symptoms, and serology is only a second line, supplementary test for supporting the clinical diagnosis (CDC, 1997). Moreover, guidelines also emphasize that serological confirmation does not need in cases of characteristic symptoms (e.g. EM). The bigger half of the Lb patients belongs to this group. Beyond EM, there are only very few patients whom pretest probability high for positive result of Bb antibody testing. For example, lymphocytic meningoradiculitis (LMR) with high protein and low glucose level in the CSF (Lakos, 1992), and facial palsy becoming bilateral in two weeks or with a tick bite behind the auricle are very suspicious for Bb infection (Lakos, unpublished), as well as fluctuating arthritis of the knee with impressive swelling but relatively moderate pain (Gerster et al., 1981; Shapiro & Gerber, 2000).

The number of these patients with high pretest probability is dwarfed by the total number of suspect cases. Oligoarthritis can be caused by many other illnesses, the etiology of facial palsy is also divers. In most of the LMR cases the stiff neck is minimal (Ryberg, 1984; Sindic et al., 1987); therefore cerebrospinal fluid exam is rarely done. Moreover, most of the LMR patients are treated with antibiotics before the suspicion of Lb would arise, and this may abort the antibody response. Chronic Borrelia meningitis is rarely seen in the last decade. In spite of the guidelines' advice, most of the Bb antibody tests are done in the patients with low pretest probability for positive Bb antibody result (Coumou et al., 2011; Lakos et al., 2010).

The basic problem is that where the (i) pretest probability is high, evaluation of the clinical signs (e.g. EM) is more sensitive than serology, therefore antibody testing is not warranted, while in cases (ii) with low pretest probability (e.g. general symptoms, malaise, fatigue, polyneuropathy, arthralgia, myalgia) is again contraindicated just because of the low PPV (Lakos et al., 2010, Lakos & Igari, 2011). Following these rules, there would be a very few cases where Bb antibody test is reasonable. Why are so many tests done after all?

Half of the adult population complains of some kind of musculoskeletal symptoms in a nationwide US prevalence study (Lawrence et al., 2008). This means that Bb antibody testing may need with reason in everyone at least once in a period of life. Moreover, patients and their doctors would like to change the diagnosis of an incurable disease (e.g., multiple sclerosis, rheumatoid arthritis) to a curable one (i.e., Lb) or a disease of unknown origin to a disease with a clear-cut etiology. Therefore, there is a strong pressure on doctors to test for Bb antibodies in patients suffering from diseases of serious course and/or of unknown origin. This pressure leads to the substantial consumption of Bb antibody tests. Only at the Mayo Clinic more than 75.000 tests were done in a year (Binnicker et al., 2008). The more tests are consumed the more false positive results are expected.

If the clinical sign is not typical for Lb, a single positive serological result must not be accepted as a proof of Bb infection and must not be followed by antibiotic treatment. Instead, a second sample should be drawn after an interval, and then not the positivity but the tendency of the antibody production, i.e. presence or absence of the progression will provide definitive result and strong support for the clinician whether the treatment is indicated or not. Applying COMPASS in those cases where the clinical signs are not typical for Lb may decrease the false diagnoses and antibiotic abuse.

Only Wb is appropriate for the comparative test, since progression in one or two antibodies can be faded by the total amount of antibody response. (ELISA measures the whole amount of antibodies; therefore only massive difference between the sample pair may be evaluable with this method). Parallel examination of the sample pair is also important since the intralaboratory fluctuation of the results can be more intense than the real change in the patient.

5. Summary

COMPASS

a. May help the clinician in cases suspicious for EM but the clinical diagnosis is not clean cut. A blood sample should be drawn at the first visit, and if the rash does not develop into a typical form, wait for collecting the second sample instead of antibiotic treatment. Than the sample pair is examined in parallel and the presence / absence of the progression provide a definitive judgment whether the patient acquired Bb infection or not.
b. It is useful for proving the microbiological cure.

c. It is useful for determining the diagnosis when the first sample reveals positive antibody response but the clinical symptoms are not specific for Lb.
d. It is appropriate for the demonstration of the intrathecal Borrelia antibody production. In this setting the assay is completed with serum and CSF pair drawn at the same day (Lakos et al., 2005).
e. It is useful in distinguishing present and past Bb infection in high risk group patients (forestry workers, orienteers, hunters, etc.) where the positive serological reaction is quite frequent but Lb with clinical symptoms is relatively rare (Lakos 2011).
f. It is appropriate for proof /exclusion of the persistent, relapsed and repeated infections.
g. It may be appropriate for comparison of different antibiotic treatment / regime in such a disease (i.e. EM) where the spontaneous clinical improvement is frequent.
h. It is probably appropriate for disclosing materno-fetal transmission of Bb in cases of Lb during pregnancy.

COMPASS would probably help in other infection where serology is routinely applied but present and past infection can not be distinguished easily (e.g. Toxoplasma gondii, Chlamydophila pneumoniae etc.).

6. References

Ackermann, R.; Hörstrup, P. & Schmidt, R. (1984). Tick-borne meningoneuritis (Garin-Bajadoux, Bannwarth). *The Yale Journal of Biology and Medicine,* Vol.57, No.4, (July-August 1984), pp. 485-490

Andrew, M. A.; Easterling, T. R.; Carr, D. B; Shen, D.; Buchanan, M. L.; Rutherford, T; Bennett, R.; Vicini, P. & Herbert, M. F. (2007). Amoxicillin pharmacokinetics in pregnant women: modeling and simulations of dosage strategies. *Clinical Pharmacology and Therapeutics,* Vol.81, No.4, (April 2007), pp. 547–556

Ang, C.W.; Notermans, D.W.; Hommes, M.; Simoons-Smit, A. & Herremans, T. (2011). Large differences between test strategies for the detection of anti-Borrelia antibodies are revealed by comparing eight ELISAs and five immunoblots. *European Journal of Clinical Microbiology & Infectious Diseases,* Vol.30, No.8, (August 2011), pp. 1027-1032

Arnez, M.; Pleterski-Rigler, D.; Luznik-Bufon, T.; Ruzić-Sabljić, E. & Strle, F. (2002). Solitary erythema migrans in children: comparison of treatment with azithromycin and phenoxymethylpenicillin. *Wiener Klinische Wochenschrift,* Vol.114, No.13-14, (July 2002), pp. 498-504

Ashburn, D.; Davidson, M. M.; Joss, A. W.; Pennington, T. H. & Ho-Yen, D. O. (1998). Improved diagnosis of reactivated toxoplasmosis. *Molecular Pathology,* Vol.51, No.2, (April 1998), pp.105-109

Bacon, R.M.; Biggerstaff, B.J.; Schriefer, M.E.; Gilmore, R.D. Jr; Philipp, M.T..; Steere, A.C.; Wormser, G.P.; Marques, A.R. & Johnson, B.J. (2003). Serodiagnosis of Lyme disease by kinetic enzyme-linked immunosorbent assay using recombinant VlsE1 or peptide antigens of Borrelia burgdorferi compared with 2-tiered testing using whole-cell lysates. *The Journal of Infectious Diseases,* Vol.187, No.8, (April 2003), pp. 1187–99

Banyas, G. T. (1992). Difficulties with Lyme serology. *Journal of the American Optometric Associaion,* Vol.63, No.2, (February 1992), pp. 135-139

Baradaran-Dilmaghani, R. & Stanek, G. (1996). In vitro susceptibility of thirty Borrelia strains from various sources against eight antimicrobial chemotherapies. *Infection*, Vol.24, No.1, (January-February 1996), pp. 60–63

Binnicker, M.J.; Jespersen, D.J.; Harring, J.A.; Rollins, L.O.; Bryant, S.C. & Beito, E. M. (2008). Evaluation of two commercial systems for automated processing, reading, and interpretation of Lyme borreliosis Western blots. *Journal of Clinical Microbiology*, Vol.46, No.7, (July 2008), pp. 2216-2221

Burgdorfer, W.; Barbour, A. G.; Hayes, S. F.; Benach, J. L.; Grunwaldt, E. & Davis, J. P. (1982). Lyme disease-a tick-borne spirochetosis? *Science*, Vol.216, No.4552, (June 1982), pp. 1317-1319

Coumou, J.; van der Poll, T.; Speelman, P. & Hovius, J.W. (2011). Tired of Lyme borreliosis. Lyme borreliosis in the Netherlands. *The Netherlands Journal of Medicine*, Vol.69, No.3, (March 2011), pp. 101-111

Centers for Disease Control and Prevention. (1995). Recommendations for Test Performance and Interpretation from the Second National Conference on Serologic Diagnosis of Lyme Disease. *MMWR Morbidity and Mortality Weekly Report*, Vol.44, No.31, (August 1995), pp. 590-591

Centers for Disease Control and Prevention. (1997). Case definitions for infectious conditions under public health surveillance. *MMWR Recommandations and Reports*, Vol.46, No.10, (May 1997), pp. 1-55

Centers for Disease Control and Prevention. (2008). Lyme Disease (Borrelia burgdorferi) 2008 Case definition. In: www.cdc.gov, 01.09.2011, Available from: http://www.cdc.gov/osels/ph_surveillance/nndss/casedef/lyme_disease_2008.htm

Craft, J. E.; Grodzicki, R. L.; Shrestha, M.; Fischer, D. K.; García-Blanco, M. & Steere, A. C. (1984). The antibody response in Lyme disease. *The Yale Journal of Biology and Medicine*, Vol.57, No.4, (July-August 1984), pp. 561-565

Cutler, S. J. & Wright, D. J. (1994). Predictive value of serology in diagnosing Lyme borreliosis. *Journal of Clinical Pathology*, Vol.47, No.4, (April 1994), pp. 344-349

Donta, S.T. (1997). Tetracycline therapy for chronic Lyme disease. *Clinical Infectious Diseases*, Vol.25, Suppl.1, (July 1997), pp. 52-56

Dressler, F.; Whalen, J. A.; Reinhardt, B. N. & Steere, A. C. (1993). Western blotting in the serodiagnosis of Lyme disease. *The Journal of Infectious Diseases*, Vol.167, No.2, (February 1993), pp. 392–400

Gerster, J. C.; Guggi, S.; Perroud, H. & Bovet, R. (1981). Lyme arthritis appearing outside the United States: a case report of Switzerland. *British Medical Journal*, Vol.283, No.6297, (October 1981), pp. 951-952

Goettner, G.; Schulte-Spechtel, U.; Hillermann, R.; Liegl, G.; Wilske, B. & Fingerle, V. (2005). Improvement of Lyme borreliosis serodiagnosis by a newly developed recombinant immunoglobulin G (IgG) and IgM line immunoblot assay and addition of VlsE and DbpA homologues. *Journal of Clinical Microbiology*. Vol.43, No.8, (August 2005), pp. 3602-3609

Halperin, J. J., Volkman, D. J. & Wu, P. (1991). Central nervous system abnormalities in Lyme neuroborreliosis. *Neurology*, Vol.41, No.10, (October 1991), pp. 1571-1582

Hauser, U.; Lehnert, G.; Lobentanzer, R. & Wilske, B. (1997). Interpretation criteria for standardized Western blots for three European species of Borrelia burgdorferi sensu lato. *Journal of Clinical Microbiology*, Vol.35, No.6, (June 1997), pp. 1433-1444

Hunfeld, K. P.; Ruzic-Sabljic, E.; Norris, D. E.; Kraiczy, P. & Strle, F. (2005). In vitro susceptibility testing of Borrelia burgdorferi sensu lato isolates cultured from patients with erythema migrans before and after antimicrobial chemotherapy. *Antimicrobial Agents and Chemotherapy,* Vol.49, No.5, (April 2005), pp. 1294-1301

Kaiser, R. (2000). False-negative serology in patients with neuroborreliosis and the value of employing of different borrelial strains in serological assays. *Journal of Medical Microbiology,* Vol.49, No.10, (October 2000), pp. 911-915

Kannian, P.; McHugh, G.; Johnson, B. J.; Bacon, R. M.; Glickstein, L. J. & Steere, A. C. (2007). Antibiotic responses to Borrelia burgdorferi in patients with antibiotic-refractory, antibiotic-responsive, or non-antibiotic-treated Lyme arthritis. *Arthritis and Rheumatism,* Vol.56, No.12, (December 2007), pp. 4216-4225

Karlsson, M.; Hammers, S; Nilsson-Ehle, I.; Malmborg, A. S. & Wretlind, B. (1996) Concentrations of doxycycline and penicillin G in sera and cerebrospinal fluid of patients treated for neuroborreliosis. *Antimicrobial Agents and Chemotherapy,* Vol.40, No.5, (May 1996), pp. 1104-1107

Kleibeuker, W.; Zhou, X.; Centlivre, M.; Legrand, N.; Page, M.; Almond, N.; Berkhout, B. & Das, A. T. (2009) A sensitive cell-based assay to measure the doxycycline concentration in biological samples. *Human Gene Therapy,* Vol.20, No.5 (May 2009), pp. 524-530

Klempner, M. S.; Hu, L. T.; Evans, J.; Schmid, C. H.; Johnson, G. M.; Trevino, R. P.; Norton, D.; Lew, L.; Wall, D.; McCall, J.; Kosinksi, M. & Weinstein, A. (2001). Two controlled trials of antibiotic treatment in patients with persistent symptoms and a history of Lyme disease. *The New England Journal of Medicine,* Vol.45, No.2, (July 2001), pp. 85–92

Lakos, A. (1990). Comparison of four serological tests for Borrelia burgdorferi in Bell's palsy. *Seroiagnosis and Immunotherapy,* Vol.4, No.4, (August 1990), pp. 271-275

Lakos, A. (1992). Cerebrospinal findings in Lyme meningitis. *The Journal of Infection,* Vol.25, No.2, (September 1992), pp. 1-12

Lakos, A. & Granström, M. (1997). Diagnostic power of immunoblot in Lyme borreliosis. *Proceedings of The 15th Annual meeting of the European Society for Paediatric Infectious Disease,* Paris, France, May, 1997

Lakos, A.; Ferenczi, E.; Komoly, S. & Granström, M. (2005). Different B-cell populations are responsible for the peripheral and intrathecal antibody production in neuroborreliosis. *International Immunology,* Vol.17, No.12, (December 2005), pp. 1631-1637

Lakos, A.; Nagy, G. & Deák, L. C. (2008). Evaluation of the serological progression (COMPASS) in Lyme borreliosis (Hungarian). *Medicus Anonymus,* Vol.16, No.5-6. (May 2008), pp.20-21

Lakos, A. & Solymosi, N. (2010). Maternal Lyme borreliosis and pregnancy outcome. *The International Journal of Infectious Diseases,* Vol.14, No.6, (June 2010), pp. e494-498

Lakos, A.; Reiczigel, J. & Solymosi, N. (2010). The positive predictive value of Borrelia burgdorferi serology in the light of symptoms of patients sent to an outpatient service for tick-borne diseases. *Inflammation Research,* Vol.59, No.11, (November 2010), pp. 959-964

Lakos, A. & Igari, E. (2011). Clinical and serological survey for Lyme borreliosis among forestry workers (Hungarian). *Háziorvos Továbbképző Szemle,* Vol.16, (2011), pp. 10-12

Lawrence, R.C.; Felson, D.T.; Helmick, C.G.; Arnold, L.M.; Choi, H.; Deyo, R.A.; Gabriel, S.; Hirsch, R.; Hochberg, M.C.; Hunder, G.G.; Jordan, J.M.; Katz, J.N.; Kremers, H.M. & Wolfe, F. (National Arthritis Data Workgroup). (2008). Estimates of the prevalence of arthritis and other rheumatic conditions in the United States. *Arthritis and Rheumatism,* Vol.58, No.1, (January 2008), pp. 26–35

Marangoni, A.; Sparacino, M.; Cavrini, F.; Storni, E.; Mondardini, V.; Sambri, V. & Cevenini, R. (2005). Comparative evaluation of three different ELISA methods for the diagnosis of early culture-confirmed Lyme disease in Italy. *Journal of Clinical Microbiology,* Vol.54, No.4, (April 2005), pp. 361-367

Maraspin, V.; Lotric-Furlan, S. & Strle, F. (2002). Development of erythema migrans in spite of treatment with antibiotics after a tick bite. *Wiener Klinische Wochenschrift,* Vol.114, No.13-14, (July 2002), pp. 616-619

Marques, A. (2008). Chronic Lyme disease: a review. *Infectious Disease Clinics of North America,* Vol.22, No.2, (June 2008), pp. 341-360

Nohlmans, M. K.; Blaauw, A. A.; van den Bogaard, A. E. & van Boven, C. P. (1994). Evaluation of nine serological tests for diagnosis of Lyme borreliosis. *Europian Jounal of Clinical Microbiology and Infectious Diseases,* Vol.13, No.5, (May 1994), pp. 394-400

Numthavaj, P.; Thakkinstian, A.; Dejthevaporn, C. & Attia, J. (2011). Corticosteroid and antiviral therapy for Bell's palsy: a network meta-analysis. *BMC Neurology,* Vol.11, (January 2011), pp. 1

Pachner, A. R. & Steere, A. C. (1984). Neurological findings of Lyme disease. *The Yale Journal of Biology and Medicine,* Vol.57, No.4, (July-August 1984), pp. 481-483

Porwancher, R.B.; Hagerty, C.G.; Fan, J.; Landsberg, L.; Johnson, B.J.; Kopnitsky, M.; Steere, A.C.; Kulas, K. & Wong, S.J. (2011). Multiplex immunoassay for Lyme disease using VlsE1-IgG and pepC10-IgM antibodies: improving test performance through bioinformatics. *Clinical and Vaccine Immunology,* Vol.18, No.5, (May 2011), pp. 851-859

Raoult, D., Hechemy, K. E. & Baranton, G. (1989). Cross-reaction with Borrelia burgdorferi antigen of sera from patients with human immunodeficiency virus infection, syphilis, and leptospirosis. *Journal of Clinical Microbiology,* Vol.27, No.10, (October 1989), pp. 2152-2155

Rath, P. M.; Marsch, W. C., Brade, V. & Fehrenbach, F. (1994). Serological distinction between syphilis and Lyme borreliosis. *Zentralblatt für Mikrobiologie,* Vol.280, No.3, (January 1994), pp. 319-324

Robertson, J.; Guy, E.; Andrews, N.; Wilske, B.; Anda, P.; Granström, M., Hauser, U.; Moosmann, Y; Sambri, V.; Schellekens, J. & Stanek, G. (2000). A European multicenter study of immunoblotting in serodiagnosis of Lyme borreliosis. *Journal of Clinical Microbiology,* Vol.38, No.6, (June 2000), pp. 2097–2102

Ryberg, B. (1984). Bannwarth's syndrome (lymphocytic meningoradicultis) in Sweden. *The Yale Journal of Biology and Medicine.* Vol.57, No.4, (July-August 1984), pp. 499-503

Shapiro, E. D. & Gerber, M. A. (2000). Lyme disease. *Clinical Infectious Disease,* Vol.31, No.2, (August 2000), pp. 533-542

Sindic, C. J.; Depre, A.; Bigaigon, G.; Goubau, P., F.; Hella, P. & Laterre, C. (1987). Lymphocytic meningoradiculitis and encephalomyelitis due to Borrelia burgdorferi: a clinical and serological study of 18 cases. *Journal of Neurology, Neurosurgery, and Psychiatric.* Vol.50, No.12, (December 1987), pp. 1565-1571

Stanek G, O'Connell S, Cimmino M, Aberer E, Kristoferitsch W, Granström M, Guy E, Gray J. (1996). European Union Concerted Action on Risk Assessment in Lyme Borreliosis: clinical case definitions for Lyme borreliosis. *Wiener Klinische Wochenschrift,* Vol.108, No.23, (December, 1996), pp.741-747.),

Stanek, G. & Strle, F. (2003). Lyme borreliosis. *Lancet,* Vol.362, No.9396, (November 2003), pp. 1639-1647

Steere, A. C.; Coburn, J. & Glickstein, L. (2004). The emergence of Lyme disease. *The Journal of Clinical Investigation,* Vol.113, No.8, (April 2004), pp. 1093-1101

Steere, A. C. & Angelis, S. M. (2006). Therapy of Lyme arthritis: strategies for the treatment of antibiotic-refractory arthritis. *Arthritis and Rheumatism,* Vol.54, No.10, (October 2006), pp. 3079-3086

Steere, A.C.; McHugh, G.; Damle, N. & Sikand, V.K. (2008). Prospective study of serologic tests for Lyme disease. *Clinical Infectious Diseases,* Vol.47, No.2, (July 2008), pp.188–195

Sullivan, F. M., Swan, I. R.; Donnan, P. T., Morrison, J. M.; Smith, B. H.; McKinstry, B.; Davenport, R.J.; Vale, L. D.; Clarkson, J. E., Hammersley, V.; Hayavi, S.; McAteer, A.; Stewart, K. & Daly, F. (2007). Early treatment with prednisolone or acyclovir in Bell's palsy. *The New England Journal of Medicine,* Vol.357, No.16, (October 2007), pp. 1598-1607

Szer, I. S.; Taylor, E. & Steere, A. C. (1991). The long-term course of Lyme arthritis in children. *The New England Journal of Medicine,* Vol.325, No.3, (July 1991), pp. 159-163

Tuuminen, T.; Hedman, K.; Söderlund-Venermo, M. & Seppälä, I. (2011). Acute parvovirus B19 infection causes nonspecificity frequently in Borrelia and less often in Salmonella and Campylobacter serology, posing a problem in diagnosis of infectious arthropathy. *Clinical and Vaccine Immunology,* Vol.18, No.1, (January 2011), pp. 167-172

Wilske, B., Schierz, G., Preac-Mursic, V., von Busch, K.; Kühlbeck, R.; Pfister, H. W. & Einhäuple, K. (1986). Intrathecal production of specific antibodies against Borrelia burgdorferi in patients with lymphocytic meningoradiculitis (Bannwarth's syndrome). The Journal of Infectious Diseases, Vol.153, No.2, (February 1986), pp. 304-314

Wormser, G. P.; Ramanathan, R.; Nowakowski, J.; McKenna, D.; Holmgren, D.; Visintainer, P.; Dornbush, R.; Singh, B. & Nadelman, R. B. (2003). Duration of antibiotic therapy for early Lyme disease. A randomized, double-blind, placebo-controlled trial. *Annals of Internal Medicine,* Vol.138, No.9, (May 2003), pp. 697-704

Wormser, G. P.; Dattwyler, R. J.; Shapiro, E. D.; Halperin, J. J.; Steere, A. C.; Klempner, M. S.; Krause, P. J.; Bakken, J. S.; Strle, F.; Stanek, G.; Bockenstedt, L.; Fich, D.; Dumler, J. S. & Nadelman, R. B. (2006). The clinical assessment, treatment, and prevention of Lyme disease, human granulocytic anaplasmosis, and babesiosis: clinical practice guidelines by the Infectious Diseases Society of America. *Clinical Infectious Diseases.* Vol.43, No.9, (November 2006), pp. 1089-1134

4

The Serology Diagnostic Schemes in *Borrelia burgdorferi* Sensu Lato Infections – Significance in Clinical Practice

Małgorzata Tokarska-Rodak and Maria Kozioł-Montewka
Department of Medical Microbiology, Medical University, Lublin
Poland

1. Introduction

Lyme borreliosis is a world-wide multi-organic disease caused by spirochete *Borrelia burgdorferi* sensu lato. Numerous gene-species *Borrelia* are identified with a various frequency in Europe, Asia and America (Ruderko, et al., 2009; Siegel, et al., 2008; Stanek G, 2011; Wilske, et al., 2007 Wodecka, 2006a). Within the last few years, as well as in Europe as in North America, there were prepared strategies, directives and guidelines for diagnostics and treatment of Lyme disease, including the frequency of occurrence of specific gene-species and a specification of clinical symptoms (Center for Disease Control and Prevention [CDC], 2011; European Concerted Action on Lyme Borreliosis [EUCALB], 2008). Lyme disease seems to be easy to diagnose and treat due to the pathogenic factor known for a long-time and elaborated diagnostic and therapeutic schemas. In serological diagnostics an impediment constitutes a wide range of genospecies *B. burgdorferi,* changes of expression of particular genes occurring in various stages of an infection, and cross reactions which occur in the presence of other pathogenic microorganisms and disease entities connected with an immune response disorders. It is connected with the necessary use of appropriately configured diagnostic tests and recombinant proteins common for particular genospecies and related to the immunological response at different stages of the infection (EUCALB, 2008; Zajkowska, et al., 2006a,2006b). As well as a diagnostician as a doctor has to consider not only the results of the serological tests but also numerous, coexisting, frequently unspecified factors in order to make an accurate diagnose confirming or excluding *B. burgdorferi* infection. In many cases, even early and accurate diagnosis and antibiotic therapy appropriately applied does not guarantee the effective eradication of a pathogen, and what is important for a patient - a complete elimination of symptoms of the disease. Post-treatment Lyme disease Syndrome (PTLDS) has been confirmed in some patients – it is a complex of lingering, unspecified clinical symptoms which impede a complete physical and mental recovery in patients after being treated from Lyme disease. This is a crucial problem as well as in health as in social life which is frequently ignored. The symptoms concerning Lyme arthritis and neuroborreliosis are frequently the cause of an immense disability in patients in numerous life activities and it is required to undertake a rehabilitation program (Tokarska-Rodak et al., 2007).

2. Two-step laboratory testing process in diagnostics of Lyme disease

European Concerted Action on Lyme Borreliosis (EUCALB) and Center for Disease Control and Prevention (CDC) recommend a two-step testing process in serological diagnostics of Lyme disease (CDC, 2011; EUCALB, 2008). It has been assumed that, a diagnosis of every form of clinical disease, except erythema migrans (EM), requires the two-step testing process. The first step in the testing process uses enzyme immunoassay techniques: Indirect Immunofluorescence Assay (IFA) or Enzyme Linked Immunosorbent Assay (ELISA) in order to detect the presence of specific antibodies IgM and/or IgG (in relation to the stage of illness). ELISA or IFA tests should be confirmed by immunobloting (Western blot, Wb). In other European countries and the USA a two test procedure is recommended: a sensitive screening test such as ELISA supported by immunoblot. All specimens positive or equivocal by a ELISA or IFA should be tested by a standardized Western blot. Specimens negative by a sensitive ELISA or IFA need not by tested further. It was recommended that an IgM immunoblot be considered positive if two of the following three bands are present - OspC, (24 kDa), BmpA (39 kDa) and Flagelina (41 kDa). It was further recommended that an IgG immunoblot be considered positive if bands for antigen proteins are present: p17, p18, p21 (DbpA), OspC (p22, 23, 24, 25), OspD (p29), p30, OspA (p31), OspB (p34), p58, p83/100 and VlsE (Aberer, 2007; Deutsche Borreliose-Gesellschaft e.V, 2010; EUCALB, 2008, MMWR, 1995). Complete standardization of immunobloting protocols in Europe is unrealistic at present. Lyme borreliosis is not the same in all geographic areas due to different local prevalence of species and strains of *B. burgdorferi* s.l. and to heterogeneity within those strains. Recommendations for the interpretation of Western blots have not always been applicable to populations in geographic areas other than where they were developed. The development of immunoblots using defined recombinant or synthetic antigens is promising for the future (EUCALB, 2008; Robertson, 2000).

The test for Lyme disease (ELISA, IFA, Western blot) measures antibodies made by white blood cells in response to infection. The antibodies IgM are produced in human's body in the response against the antigen proteins *B. burgdorferi* in the 2nd-4th week since the EM exposure, reaching the ultimate in the 4th-6th week, and they are most frequently IgM anti-OspC and anti-p41. If the serological test is made too soon, it can show falsely negative results in the scope of the presence of IgM because of the low symptomatic features. Antibody response in early Lyme borreliosis may by weak or absent, especially in erythema migrans and antibiotic treatment may abrogate antibody production. Serology may also be negative in acute neuroborreliosis with short duration of the disease (EUCALB, 2008; Stanek, 2011). The repetition of Wb after 2-4 weeks should be considered in patients at an early stage in case of a positive result of an enzyme immunoassay test and negative confirmation test (Depietropaolo, et al., 2005; EUCALB, 2008; Flisiak& Pancewicz, 2011; Przytuła, et al., 2006). When Western blot is used during the first 4 weeks of disease onset (early Lyme disease), both IgM and IgG procedures should be performed (MMWR, 1995). Specific IgG and/or IgM are found in only 40-60% of untreated cases EM, particularly in patients with signs haematogenous spread (EUCALB, 2008). In most patients with an active Lyme disease, the level of the antibodies IgM decreases after about 4 months. The antibodies IgG start to emerge in a serum in the 4th week since the infection. In the early disseminated stage or the acute neuroborreliosis, the IgM/IgG seropositiveness increases 70-90%. In this period, the immunological response can be manifested in relation to few antigens. For the diagnosis

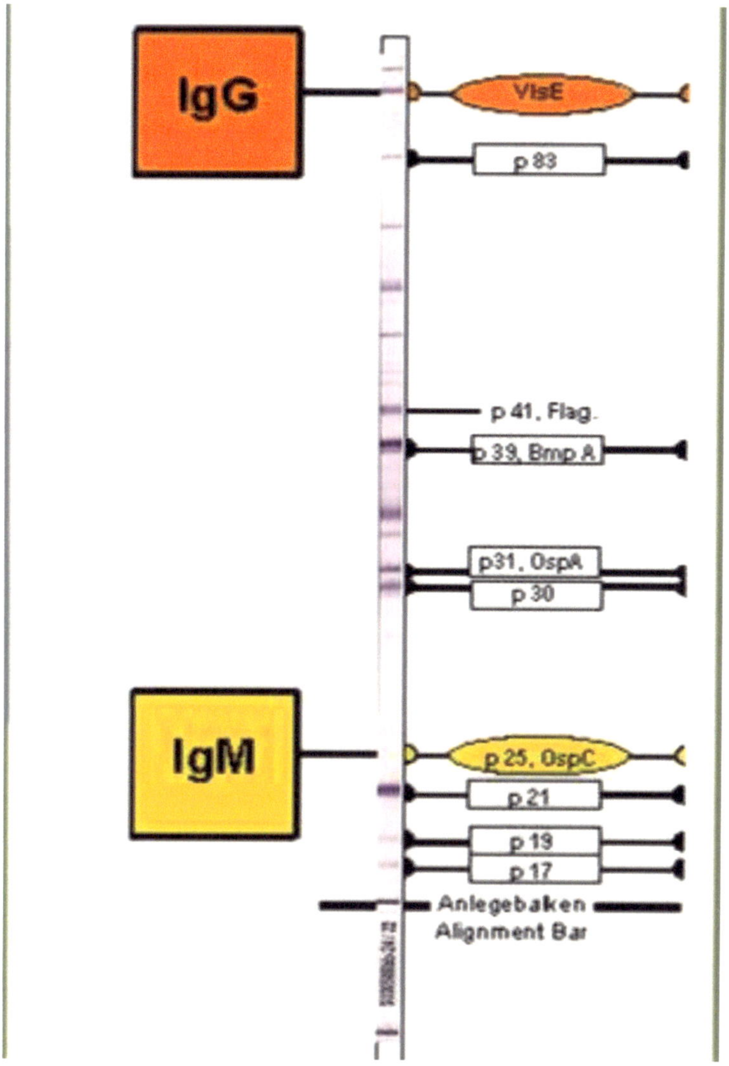

Fig. 1. Western Blot interpretation of IgM/IgG class antibodies against specific antigens plus recombinant VlsE *Borrelia burgdorferi* (according to Euroimmun).

of Lyme arthritis, it is essential to demonstrate the presence of specific IgG antibodies, usually in high levels. A positive IgM test in the absence of IgG antibodies argues against the diagnosis of Lyme arthritis. Follow-up is recommended only in cases with short duration of symptoms. For the diagnosis of acrodermatitis chronica atrophicans (ACA), it is essential to demonstrate high levels of IgG anti-*B. burgdorferi*. A positive IgM test in the absence of IgG antibodies argues against the diagnosis of ACA (EUCALB, 2008). Technical problems that contribute to false-negative or false-positive results include the adoption of inadequate cut-off levels, the presence of cross-reacting antibodies, false positive reactions caused by some autoimmune diseases and inappropriate interpretation criteria for Western blots (Stanek, 2011). Results are considered positive only if the ELISA/IFA and the immunoblot are both positive. CDC does not recommended skipping the first test and just doing the Western blot. Doing so will increase the frequency of false positive results and may lead to misdiagnosis and improper treatment (CDC, 2011). According to the directives, which are mandatory in Europe, the serological tests determining the level of antibodies IgM/IgG anti-*Borrelia burgdorferi* should not be used in the assessment of the effectiveness of the therapy. The effectiveness of the antibiotic therapy should be assessed only on the basis of the dynamics of the clinical picture (EUCALB, 2008; Flisiak & Pancewicz, 2011). It has not been defined so far that there is a parameter, which marking would reliably determine the effectiveness of the elimination of the pathogen. It has been suggested that, the decrease of the titre of the antibodies for C6 protein can be interpreted as an indicator of the effectiveness of the therapy (Aberer, 2007). The probability that a patient with a positive serological test actually has Lyme borreliosis and the probability that a patient with a negative test does not have the disease depends on the performance characteristics of a given assay (sensitivity and specificity) and also on the prevalence of the disease in the population (Stanek, 2011). Both diagnostic tests (ELISA/IFA and Wb) complement each other mutually. Serological diagnosis is always a balance between sensitivity and specificity of the assays. A high level of specificity is always more important than a high level of sensitivity (EUCALB, 2008). The enzyme immunoassay tests are characterized by high sensitivity and relatively low specificity, whereas the Wb test is characterized by high specificity and low sensitivity (Flisiak & Pancewicz, 2011). A minimum standard of a least 90% specificity for the screening tests (ELISA, IFA) and 95% specificity for the immunoblot should be established in the population where the assay is to be used (EUCALB, 2008). The two-step laboratory testing process is designed to eliminate unspecific falsely positive results which occur in a various frequency during the diagnosis with the use of one test and it allows on an explicit assessment with the interpretation of the limit results. The PCR methods are not used in a routine diagnosis of Lyme disease on account of lack of gained standards, although there are a number of researches done in this matter by many research establishments. The detection of bacteria's DNA made by the PCR method can be interpreted in two ways: it can confirm the presence of a living bacteria in an organism or it can signify on the presence of DNA coming from bacteria killed with antibiotics. The PCR method does not allow on a differentiation of DNA between living and dead being, or free DNA coming from the disintegration of the bacteria cell (Wodecka, 2006b).

3. The immunological response against the infection of *B. burgdorferi* in the aspect of clinical symptoms

The dissemination of the spirochetes into further tissues and organs occurs in a short period of time since the transmission of the infection through blood and lymphatic vessels and it is possible that through peripheral nerves as well (Sigal, 1997). The innate defense mechanisms are initiated as the first in the process of the immunological response of an organism against infection, in which as well as phagocytes as complement system, lysozyme and interferon take part. All disorders of the unspecific mechanisms in the early stage of the infection can prevent from an effective elimination of the pathogen in further stages of the immunological response, and consequently lead to the development of a chronic state of the illness (Bykowski et al., 2008; Siegel, et al., 2010). The diagnosis of the illness in patients with EM is usually made on the basis of a clinical picture without a confirmation of the serological tests, which results are frequently negative during this period. The erythema migrans usually exposes in the place of a tick's bite after 1-3 weeks. Typical EM has a form of a spot with a tendency of expanding, a diameter of more than 5 cm and a brightening in the middle. Untypical forms do not demonstrate central brightening. They can be shaped irregularly or have hemorrhagic features. The exposure of EM within the period of time shorter than 2 days after a tick's bite and of a diameter less than 5 cm oppose to the diagnosis. Erythema migrans disappear spontaneously within few days since an inception of the antibiotic therapy however it does not mean that the infection has been eliminated. The untreated lesions can stay even for few months and disappear spontaneously, though the infection still lasts (Flisiak & Pancewicz, 2011; Tokarska-Rodak, et al., 2010a, 2010b). It is essential to implement the serological test when EM takes the untypical form or does not appear and there is a suspicion of the infection with the spirochetes of *B. burgdorferi* (Zajkowska, et al. 2006). The symptoms of the disseminated Lyme disease concern: nervous system, heart, muscles and joints (Aberer, 2007; Depietropaolo, 2005). This stage of the disease appears within a few weeks till more than a year since the infection, while the late stage of Lyme disease can occur even many years after the invasion of *Borrelia* spirochetes into human body. The late stage of Lyme disease is manifested with skin lesions (acrodermatitis chronica atrophicans), chronic neurological symptoms or chronic arthritis. Borrelia arthritis can take on a chronic form leading to a permanent joint damage, and it can also be manifested by: chronic and migrating muscle pains, recurring arthritis, a pain caused by an inflammatory reaction within the scope of motor organs and the weakening of skeletal muscles (Singh, & Girschick, 2004a; Wilgat, et al., 2004). The presence of IgG for the broad antigen spectrum is observed in persons with symptoms of late Lyme disease, in 100% of patients (EUCALB, 2008; Wilske, et al., 2007). The examination of cerebrospinal fluid is made in the diagnostics of neuroborreliosis. The presence of antibodies anti-*B. burgdorferi* in the cerebrospinal fluid cannot result from their production in the cerebral space but it can be an effect of the penetration of antibodies from blood through the damaged barrier blood-brain (EUCALB, 2008). The decision concerning the diagnosis and treatment of Lyme disease is based on the clinical picture with the results of serological rests taken into account. Lyme disease should not be considered in case of the positive results of the tests and without the presence of clinical symptoms of the disease. Although, it is possible that there is a certain percentage of people in a healthy population, in whom the seropositiveness changing along with the age is observed in comparison with *B. burgdorferi* connected with outdoor activities (Bacon, et al., 2003; Wilske, et al., 2007).

4. The immunological response against *B. burgdorferi* infection in the aspect of the diversity of genospecies

There are two risk factors of acquiring infection *Borrelia* in a relation to existence on the area where the ticks are present. The first concerns the estimation of spreading *B. burgdorferi sensu lato* in ticks *Ixodes ricinus* which is the main vector of pathogen in Europe. The second factor concerns the determination of diversity of gene-species on a particular area. The risk of human infection *B. burgdorferi* s.l increases along with the number of ticks being infected on a particular area. It depends from the multiple of stabs during the haematophagy season of ticks and it becomes bigger when the time of infected ticks present on a human skin is longer (Ołdak, et al., 2009; Wodecka, 2006a). The molecular analysis has shown that isolates of *Borrelia burgdorferi* are genetically and phenotypically diversified, hence the group of species closely related of genus *Borrelia* were defined as *Borrelia burgdorferi* sensu lato. The complex of Borrelia burgdorferi sensu lato encompasses at least 12 species: B. burgdorferi sensu stricto, B. garinii, B. afzelii, B. spielmani, B. valaisiana, B. lusitaniae, B. japonica, B. andersonii, B. tunukii, B. turdae, B. bissettii and B. sinica (Aguero-Rosenfeld et al., 2005; Ruderko, et al., 2009; Sicklinger, et al., 2003; Wodecka, 2006a). According to some sources, there are also B. californiensis sp. nov. in this group (Siegel, et al., 2008). B. afzelii, B. garinii, B. burgdorferi sensu stricto and occasionally B. spielmani, B. valaisiana, B. lusitaniae are responsible for causing Lyme disease in Europe whereas in South America only B. burgdorferi sensu stricto (Siegel, et al., 2008; Stanek G, 2011; Wilske, et al., 2007). Even though Lyme disease is most generally caused in Europe by the above mentioned three genospecies Borrelia, it cannot be excluded that there are other genospecies causing the symptoms of the disease. DNA of B. valaisiana was detected in the cerebrospinal fluid of a patient with chronic neuroborreliosis in Greece and in a patient with erythema migrans. B. lusitaniae was isolated from a patient with suspected Lyme disease in Portugal (Derdáková & Lenčáková, 2005). Direct relation of skin changes of erythema migrans (EM) type with an infection of B. spielmani was revealed in some of the European countries (Netherlands, Germany, Hungary, Slovenia). Thus, the relation of these gene-species with Lyme disease has been proven (Maraspin, 2006; Wilske, et al., 2007). The genetic changeability of Borrelia has an influence as well as on the spirochetes' pathogenicity as on the clinical manifestations of the disease. Consequently, the heterogeneity of microorganisms causing Lyme disease in Europe should be taken into consideration in the serological and microbiological diagnostics (Derdáková & Lenčáková, 2005; Richter et al., 2004; Wang et al., 1999; Wilske, et al., 2007). It has been proven that Borrelia afzelii is responsible for skin lesions of type acrodermatitis chronica athropicans (ACA) and the presence of borrelia lymphocytoma, whereas B. garinii has been isolated more frequently from the cerebrospinal fluid and thus its relation with neuroborreliosis is emphasized. B. burgdorferi s.s. is responsible for lesions type arthritis. As well as the late skin lesions as neuroborreliosis are more often detected in Europe whereas Lyme arthritis is more often diagnosed in the USA (Derdáková & Lenčáková, 2005, Wilske, et al., 2003, 2007). All three genospecies *B. burgdorferi* s.s., *Borrelia afzelii* and *Borrelia garinii* can participate in the development of erythema migrans. However, there are differences present in the clinical manifestation of EM caused by those genospecies (Maraspin, 2006; Wodecka, 2006a). According to the serological diagnostics, it is essential to notice whether antibodies IgM/IgG, which are produced in the autoimmune response against the infection caused by other genospecies than those three known as pathogenic in Europe, can be detected by diagnostic tests used in a standard diagnostics of Lyme disease. The problem, among many other things, concerns infections caused only by B. spielmani. The results showing that there is a possibility of the infection caused by few genospecies B. burgdorferi s.l. has been obtained in the analysis of the presence of antibodies for antigen proteins OspC and p18 of four genospecies B. burgdorferi s.s., B. afzelii, B. garinii and B. spielmani in patients with symptoms of Lyme arthritis from Eastern Poland (Tokarska-Rodak, et al., 2010c). The identification of antibodies anti- OspC B. spielmani seems to be extremely important considering previous stage of immunological answer when only antibodies IgM anti-OspC are frequently present without antibodies of IgG class. In the case of infection with only one gene-species, the identification of antibodies IgM anti-OspC can be the only chance in the early identification of the infection with the lack of skin symptoms as EM. Diagnostic tests used routinely in the Lyme disease diagnosis in Europe (ELISA, Western blot) usually have antigen extracts of B. burgdorferi s.s., B. afzelii, B. garinii or electrophoreticaly separated antigen extracts of Borrelia afzelii enriched with recombinant VlsE antigen. According to researchers, the antigens B. spielmani - gene-species, which researchers mentioned as the fourth next to B. burgdorferi s.s., B. afzelii, B. garinii, should be additionally used in the tests and be considered in the diagnosis of Lyme disease within Europe (Derdáková & Lenčáková, 2005; Maraspin, 2006; Tokarska-Rodak, et al., 2010c).

4.1 The antigen proteins *B. burgdorferi* diagnostically significant

In the clinical practice the evaluation of the active stage of infection is primarily based on the clinical symptomatology, routine enzyme immunoassays, and confirmatory tests such as Western Blot (CDC, 2011; Štefančikowá, et al., 2005; Tokarska-Rodak, et al., 2010a). The identification of the antibodies IgM and IgG directed against specific antigenic proteins *B. burgdorferi* constitutes the basis of the serological diagnostics of Lyme disease. It becomes essential in Europe to use tests with appropriately selected antigenic panel considering the heterogeneity of the proteins *Borrelia burgdorferi* (Štefančiková, et al., 2005). The evolution of a production of the antibodies directed against various antigens *B. burgdorferi* is observed along with the development of the disease process after the transmission of the spirochetes into human body. In the early stage of the infection (2 to 4 weeks) the immunological system detects only few antigens *Borrelia* as p41 (flagellin) and proteins Osp and produces the antibodies IgM against them. OspC is an immunogenic lipoprotein and main virulent factor of the infection in people (particularly genotypes OspC A, B, I, K). OspC poorly succumbs to an expression in a tick's bowels and in a cultivation, however it undergoes intensively only after the transmission of a spirochete into a mammal organism. OspC and OspA are the most important proteins of the outer membrane in the cell of *B. burgdorferi*. OspC is characterized by large polymorphism and a substantial reactivity in comparison with OspA. Both antigens are connected with genetic and antigen heterogeneity among various species. The classification is made on the basis of various genotypes or serotypes. There have been 8 different serotypes OspA and 16 serotypes OspC (*B. burgdorferi* s.s 6 serotypes, *B. afzelii* 4 serotypes, *B. garinii* 6 serotypes) registered in Europe (Aberer, 2007; Wodecka, 2006a). The surface proteins of a spirochete affect significant stages of the immunological response: OspA inhibits the spirochetes' phagocytosis and an oxygen explosion in neutrophils especially at the low concentration of a complement, which substantially simplifies the survival and the dissemination of bacteria. The spirochetes can bind with the receptor cells molecules of a host and the extracellular matrix as integrins, glycoproteins, and proteoglycans (Hartiala, et al., 2008). The antibodies IgG anti-*B. burgdorferi* appears after several weeks since the bite, and their level can remain increased and continue even after the resolution of the clinical symptoms. As far as the infection develops, the immunologic response extends on the increasing number of antigen proteins –p83, p58, p53, p43, p39, BBK32 (p35), p31, p30 (OspA), p25 (OspC), p21, p19, DbpA (p17). The recombinant antigens OspC, p100, VlsE, DbpA (p17), BBK32p66, peptides C10 and C6 are used in order to improve the diagnostics of Lyme disease and for a better prediction of the duration of the infection (Aberer, 2007; Aguero-Rosenfeld et al., 2005; Tokarska-Rodak, et al., 2008, 2010a; Wilske, et al., 2007). The selected antigens such as p83/100, BmpA (p39) or antigens of high specificity but common for many microorganisms (e.g. the protein of flagellum- flagellin) are introduced. Flagellin (p41) is one of the most immunogenic protein which occurs in the cell of *B. burgdorferi* and causes very strong and early humoral response. Epitopes, which are characteristic for *B. burgdorferi,* only occur between 129 and 251 aminoacid. The protein which comes from the initial and final part of the chain shows a high degree of the homology with the sequence of flagellin's aminoacids *Bacillus subtilis* (65%) and *Salmonella Typhimurium* (56%). The use of the parts only specific for *B. burgdorferi* in diagnostic tests has an influence on the decrease of the percentage of results falsely positive, especially for IgM (Aguero-Rosenfeld, et al., 2005). Other sensitive and specific antigen which may be used in the serological confirmation of the infection is DbpA (p17). Its presence was confirmed in 93% of patients with Lyme arthritis and in 100% of patients with neuroborreliosis (Aberer, 2007). As indicated by the diagnostics of infections caused by *B. burgdorferi* s. l., the essential antigens are highly immunogenic proteins developing in vivo after the spirochetes' transmission into human body. The antigens VlsE, BBA 36 (22kDa), BBO 323 (42 kDa), Crasp 3 (21 kDa), pG (22 kDa) show the expression in vivo and contain highly immunogenic epitopes common for *B. burgdorferi* sensu lato, which are an important determinant for an advanced stages of Lyme disease in the serology of IgG (Bykowski, et al., 2007; Hofmann, et al., 2006; Tokarska-Rodak, et al., 2010a, Wilske, et al., 2007, Zajkowska et al., 2006b). The researchers believe VlsE protein is the most sensitive recombinated *B. burgdorferi* s.l. antigen used in the diagnostics. It is possible to detect IgM/IgG anty-VlsE in all pathogenic *Borrelia burgdorferi* sensu lato genospecies and the risk of false positive results is ten times lower in comparison to other *Borrelia* antigens (Chmielewska-Badora et al., 2006, Liang et al., 2000, Wilske, et al., 2007). In spite of an advanced stage of Lyme disease in some patients, there can be the continuity of the antibodies IgM in relation to the outer superficial protein OspC and VlsE (Hofmann, 2006, Tokarska-Rodak, 2010a). As far as antigen VlsE currently occurs in mostly used serological test ELISA and Western blot, the other antigens are not included into routine diagnostics. There are highly immunogenic proteins CRASPs (complement regulator-acquiring surface proteins) found beside antigen VlsE during the infection of *B. burgdorferi* e.g. CRASP-3, proteins belonging to Erp family (pG), and lots of membrane proteins (immunogenic membrane-associated proteins) among which there is BBO323 (Nowak, et al., 2006; Singh & Girschick, 2004a). The researches confirm the significance of the antigens in vivo in the immunological response against the infection *B. burgdorferi.* The researches conducted by Hofmann and his associates shown that antigens BBA36, BBO323, Crasp3, pG are characteristic for the late infections of Borrelia. It has been confirmed that there are the antibodies IgG for BBO323 (90%), BBA36 (67%), p83 (71%) in patients with Lyme arthritis but very seldom antibodies for Crasp3 (38%) and pG (33%) (Hofmann, et al., 2006). The presence of the antibodies IgG anty–VlsE, Crasp3, BBO323, BBA36 has been confirmed with various frequency in patients bitten many times by ticks and with clinical manifestation of Lyme arthritis (Tokarska-Rodak, et al., 2008, 2010a). The presence of antibodies IgG for VlsE and BBO323 have also been confirmed in persons being suspected of the disease, who had erythema migrans (Zajkowska, et al., 2006a, 2006b). It has been assumed that, the routine use of a broaden spectrum of the antigens in vivo (beside VlsE) in Western blot tests can contribute to the designation of the severity and dynamics of the immunological response against the used antigens, what will provide more possibilities in the assessment of the immune reactions in relation to a clinical state of a patient.

5. The immunological factors essential in the response of a hosts' organism against the infection of *B. burgdorferi*

In the light of the current knowledge, some diseases and infections are started to be considered in the aspect of probable disfunctions in the control of functioning of the elements of immunological system, including complement system. It allows to look from a different perspective on many disease entities, which are caused by infections of particular pathogenic microorganisms (Klaska, & Nowak, 2007).

5.1 The complement system

The dissemination of spirochetes Borrelia in the human organism and the development of the infection is a complex, omnidirectional process which occurs owing to many adjustments and mechanisms allowing bacteria to survive. It seems to be essential that *B. burgdorferi* is able to avoid destructive effect of the congenital defence mechanisms. The complement system participates in the elimination of *B. Burgdorferi,* and its activation on the surface of the pathogen leads to the cytolitical damage of bacteria (Bykowski, et al., 2007). The disactivation of activation cascades of the complement allows *Borrelia* to survive and also determines a competent reservoir for particular genospecies of bacteria (Siegel, et al., 2010). There are also other microorganisms apart from *Borrelia burgdorferi,* like: *Echinococcus granulosus, Neisseria meningitidis, Neisseria gonorrhoeae, Streptococcus pyogenes, Streptococcus pneumoniae, Yersinia enterocolitica, Candida albicans* and human immunodeficiency viruses which have developed mechanisms allowing to overcome the destructive process of the complement system. The acquisition of regulatory molecules of a host allows to avoid an adverse effect of the complement (Klaska, & Nowak, 2007). The microorganisms bind the human fluid phase complement regulators factor H or FHL-1 and some also bind the clasical pathway regulator C4Bp directly to the surface (Krajczy, et al., 2001). Precise analysis *in vitro* within many isolates of three pathogenic genospecies *Borrelia burgdorferi* s.l. shown that all isolates of the same genospecies have similar sensitivity on the complement's effect, however there are significant differences among genospecies. The isolates of *B. afzelii* are particularly resistant to the complement's effect, the majority of *B. burgdorferi* s.s. isolates are on average sensitive, whereas *B. garinii* are fundamentally sensitive on the effect of the complement system (Suchonen, et al., 2002). It is well known that *B. burgdorferi* s.s B31, which come from North America, are less sensitive on the complement's effect than those which come from Europe. The difference comes from a various capacity to bind component C9, which as a result leads to the reduction of the living functions of the spirochetes, and morphological changes and the fragmentation of a bacteria cell (Krajczy, et al., 2001). Proteins CRASPs (Complement Regulator - Acquiring Surface Proteins) are responsible for the ability to disactivate the complement in the case of *Borrelia burgdorferi* s.l., which are able to bind regulatory proteins of an alternative way, and as a result have an influence on the inhibition of the activation cascade of the complement. CRASPs (from CRASP-1 to CRASP-5) are connected with the soluble forms of the two regulatory proteins - factor H and factor H-like protein 1 (FHL-1) and hence the activation of the complement on the surface of bacteria does not occur. A lot of strains of *B. afzelii* and some of *B. burgdorferi* s.s. are capable to control the alternative way of the complement through the absorption of FHL-1 and H molecules. That kind of capability does not have *B. garinii* which are sensitive on the complement's effect (Krajczy, et al., 2001; Suchonen, et al., 2002; Zajkowska, et al., 2006c). Serum resistance of B. burgdorferi B31 is mainly associated witch CRASP-1 and mediated by binding of complement regulator factor H. OspA and OspC do not bind factor H (Hartiala, et al., 2008). Regardless of the way on which the activation of the complement occurs, the development of the membrane - attack complex (MAC) is a key stage. The researches indisputably confirmed the significance of the complement in the bacteriolysis of Borrelia. The spirochetes induce oxidative burst and calcium mobilization and are susceptible to phagocytosis dependent on the complement (Suchonen, et al., 2000, 2002; Krajczy, et al., 2001). The lack of susceptibility to the effect of the mechanisms of innate immunity, end especially the immunity on the destruction with the use of the complement, is determined as the virulent factor of Borrelia burgdorferi (Siegel, et al., 2010).

5.2 Lyme disease in the aspect of the autoimmunological processes

The researchers name the long duration of the disease as one of the risk factors of the occurrence of *Borreliosis* which is not curable. One cannot exclude the possibility that the long lasting infection of *B. burgdorferi,* next to typical symptoms of Lyme disease, may also induce the autoimmunological changes in a small percent of patients. The autoimmunological processes can contribute to maintain excessive inflammatory response in late Lyme disease and can be responsible for the inflammatory reaction maintenance, even after the elimination of the pathogen (Grygorczuk, 2008, Kisand, 2007; Singh & Girschick, 2004b Wilgat, 2004). In certain conditions of the environmental stress, the spirochetes can undergo reversible transformation from the motile and helical into inactive, spherical cysts. That kind of forms was observed in the cerebro-spinal fluid and tissues of the patients with Lyme disease (Singh & Girschick, 2004b). The metabolically unactive alveolar forms of Borrelia (blebs forms) containing lipoproteins OspA, OspB, OspD are named as a source of long-term antigen stimulation, which lasts even during the absence of bacteria able to multiple (Stere, 2003; Śpiewak, 2004). The examination of the patients with early Lyme disease did not reveal direct connection between the presence of antibodies anti-*Borrelia* and antinuclear antibodies (ANA) (Śpiewak, 2004). It is possible that there is a relation between the initial diagnosis of Lyme disease as erythema migrans and the occurrence in the late stage in a small percentage of people, in spite of the used treatment on arthral symptoms with simultaneous presence of the antibodies ANA (Tokarska-Rodak, 2010b). According to Singh, one potential explanation for antibiotic-resistant Lyme disease is the generation of autoimmunity mediated directly or indirectly by the pathogen (Singh, & Girschick, 2004b). Apoptosis plays the most important role in the control and physiological extinguishing of the inflammatory reaction in the infections, including the infection of *B. burgdorferi.* The impairment of apoptosis of lymphocytes and other leukocytes can be connected with the risk of autoimmunization (Grygorczuk, 2008).

5.3 Problems in the diagnosis of Lyme disease are connected with the occurrence of other disease entities

There are many disease states which presence should be considered while interpreting the results of the screening tests and the confirmation tests in the direction of Lyme disease. The antibodies present in the serum of people infected with EBV, CMV or *Mycoplasma* can react crosswise with the antigens of *B. burgdorferi* e.g. p41, OspC, BmpA (p39) which direct the diagnostic proceedings in a wrong direction. The antibodies of the cross-reaction for antigens OspC, p39 *B. burgdorferi* were also observed in the samples with serum of patients with the infection *Treponema pallidum, Herpes simplex virus* (HSV) type 2 (Depietropaolo et al., 2005; Strasfeld, et al., 2005). The antigen Epstein Barr VCA-gp125 (Virus Capsid Antigen) together with antigens *B. burgdorferi* were applied in one of the WB tests used in the diagnostics of Lyme disease. Mononucleosis should be excluded in the mode of various diagnosis in the case when there is a reactivity against EBV-gp125 next to reactivity IgM against specific proteins *Borrelia.* It is widely acknowledged that in persons with autoimmune diseases carried with high index of auto-antibodies (hypergammaglobulinemia), it is necessary to consider the possibility of obtaining falsely positive results in Lyme disease serodiagnostics (EUCALB, 2008; Flisiak & Pancewicz, 2011). The denotations of the antibodies anti-*B. burgdorferi* conducted by Hofmann et al in patients with autoimmune diseases revealed a possibility of the occurrence of the cross-reaction and the obtainment of falsely positive results pointing to the existence of Lyme disease in this group of patients (Hofmann, et al., 2006). Multiple sclerosis, lupus erythematosus can give positive results, especially when the test which is used in order to determine the level of IgM anti-B. burgdorferi is based on sonicate antigens (EUCALB, 2008). Due to the growing number of people diagnosed in the direction of Lyme disease, the problem concerning the results falsely positive resulting from the cross reactions seems crucial, especially as regards to people whose symptoms of Lyme disease are unspecific and slightly intensified. Thus, in order to decrease its percentage in the largest extent, the available possibilities of diagnostics should be used.

5.4 Post - Treatment Lyme Disease Syndrome (PTLDS)

About 10-20% of patients with the diagnose of Lyme disease suffers from the clinical symptoms of constant, repeating or persistent capacity from few months to a year after the use of appropriate antibiotic therapy. The symptoms are nonspecific: muscle and joint pains, cognitive defects, increased fatigue, irritability, emotional lability, disturbances in sleep, concentration, and memory (Feder, et al., 2007). In that kind of cases, the clinical and laboratory assessment aims to exclude the possibility of treatment failure or the presence of a new condition unrelated to previous Lyme borreliosis. That kind of state is defined as post-treatment Lyme disease syndrome (PTLDS) if it is characterised by the presence of persistent symptoms syndrome and lasts longer than 6 months since the treatment. PTLDS cannot be defined as "chronic" Lyme disease, and the occurrence of the symptoms mentioned above do not justify the use of antibiotic therapy, which in these cases is useless and potentially harmful for the patient with PTLDS. The use of symptomatic treatment is recommended for the patients with PTLDS (CDC, 2011; Stanek, et al., 2011). The reason of the occurrence of PTLDS is not entirely explained. It has been assumed that lingering symptoms are due to residua damage to the tissues and immune system that occurred during the infection. Similar complications and auto-immune responses are known to occur following other infectious diseases (CDC, 2011; Seidel, et al., 2007).

6. Conclusion

Highly immunogenic proteins produced in vivo after spirochete transmission into the human body are significant antigens for the diagnostics of B. burgdorferi s.l. infections. Antigens VlsE, BBA36, BBO323 and Crasp 3 demonstrate in vivo expression and comprise highly immunogenic epitopes, common for B. burgdorferi s.l., which are important IgG serological markers of advanced stages of borreliosis. Thus a serologic test with those antigens involved creates better potential to evaluate immune response with account for clinical status of the patient. The detection of antibodies directed against specific *B. spielmani* antigens suggests that this microorganism may be responsible for triggering borreliosis both as a single etiologic agent and with other *Borrelia* genospecies. The long-lasting persistence of the disease and thus long-term antigenic stimulation can be considered as a factor enabling the initiation of autoimmune reactions. This process can exist in a small percentage of patients with Lyme disease but the possibility of its inception cannot be completely negated.

7. References

Aberer, E. (2007). Lyme borreliosis-an update. *Journal der Deutschen Dermatologischen Gesellschsft*, Vol.5, No.5, (May 2007), pp. 406-413, ISSN 1610-0387

Aguero-Rosenfeld, M. E.; Wang, G.; Schwarz, I. & Womser G.P. (2005). Diagnosis of Lyme borreliosis. *Clinical Microbiology Reviews*, Vol.18, No.3, (July 2005), pp. 484-509, ISSN 1098-6618

Bacon, R. M.; Biggerstaff, B. J. & Schriefer, M. E. (2003). Serodiagnosis of Lyme disease by kinetic enzyme-linked immunosorbent assay using recombinant VlsE or peptide antigens of Borrelia burgdorferi compared with 2-tiewred testing using whole -cell lysates. *Journal of Infectious Diseases*, Vol.187, No.8, (April 2003), pp. 1187-1199, ISSN 0022-1899

Bykowski, T.; Woodman, M. E.; Cooley, A. E. & Brisette, C. A. (2008). Borrelia burgdorferi complement regulator-acquiring surface proteins (BbCRASPs): Expression patterns during the mammal-tick infection cycle. *International Journal of Medical Microbiology*, Vol.1, No.298, Supl. 1 (September 2008), pp. 249-256, ISSN 1438-4221

Center for Disease Control and Prevention (April, 2011). Two-step Laboratory Testing Process, In: *Lyme Disease*, 20.07.2011, Available from: http://www.cdc.gov/lyme/diagnosistreatment/LabTest/TwoStep/

Chmielewska-Badora, J. Cisak, E.; Wójcik-Fatla, A.; Zwoliński, J.; Buczek, A. & Dutkiewicz, J. (2006). Correlation of tests for detection of Borrelia burgdorferi sensu lato infection in patients with diagnosed borreliosis. *Annals of Agricultural and Environmental Medicine*, Vol.13, No.2, pp. 307-311, ISSN 1232-1966

Depietropaolo, D. L.; Powers, J. H.; Gill J. M. & Foy A. J. (2005). Diagnosis of Lyme disease. *American Family Physician*, Vol.72, No.2, (July 2005), pp. 297-304, ISSN 0002-838X

Derdáková, M. & Lenčáková, D. (2005). Association of genetic variability within the Borrelia burgdorferi sensu lato with the ecology, epidemiology of Lyme borreliosis in Europe. *Annals of Agricultural and Environmental Medicine*, Vol.12, pp. 165-172, ISSN 1232-1966

Deutsche Borreliose-Gesellschaft e.V. (December, 2010) Diagnostyka i leczenie boreliozy z Lyme. Wytyczne Niemieckiego Towarzystwa Boreliozy In: *Deutsche Borreliose-Gesellschaft e.V.* 14.09.2011, Available from: http://www.borreliosegesellschaft.de/Texte/Wytyczne.pdf

European Concerted Action on Lyme Borreliosis (March, 2008). Test in use, In: *Diagnosis serology*, 20.07.2011, Available from: http://meduni09.edis.at/eucalb/cms/index.php?option=com_content&task=view&id=38&Itemid=102

Feder, H. M.; Johnson, B. J. B.; O'Connell, S.; Shapiro, E. D.; Steere, A. C.; Wormser, G. P.; & the Ad Hoc International Lyme Disease Group. A critical appraisal of "chronic Lyme disease". (2007). *The New England Journal of Medicine,* Vol.357, No.14, (October 2007), pp.1422-1430, ISSN 0028-4793

Flisiak, S. & Pancewicz, S. (July 2011). Diagnostyka i leczenie boreliozy z Lyme, In: *Zalecenia Polskiego Towarzystwa Epidemiologów i Lekarzy Chorób Zakaźnych,*19.07.2011, Available from: http://www.pteilchz.org.pl/standardy.htm

Grygorczuk, S.; Panasiuk, A.; Zajkowska, J.; Kondrusik, M.; Chmielewski, T.; Wierzbińska, R.; Pancewicz, S.; Flisiak, R. & Tylewska-Wierzbanowska, S. (2008). Activity of the caspase-3 in the culture of peripheral blood mononuclear cells stimulated with Borrelia burgdorferi antigen. *Przegląd Epidemiologiczny,* Vol.62, No.1, (2008), pp. 85-91, ISSN 0033-2100

Grygorczuk, S.; Zajkowska, J.; Kondrusik, M.; Moniuszko, A.; Pancewicz, S. & Pawlak-Zalewska, W. (2008). Failures of antibiotic treatment in Lyme arthritis. *Przegląd Epidemiologiczny,* Vol.62, No.3, (2008), pp. 581-588, ISSN 0033-2100

Hartiala, P.; Hytonen, J.; Suhonen, J.; Lepparanta, O.; Tuominen-Gustafsson, H. & Viljanen, M. K., (2008). Borrelia burgdorferi inhibits human neutrophil functions. *Microbes and Infection,* Vol.10, No.1, (January 2008), pp. 60-68, ISSN 1286-4579

Hofmann, H.; Wallich, R.; Lorenz, I. & Bechtel, M. (22 May 2006). Comparison of a new line assay using purified and recombinant antigens with a European lysate blot for serodiagnosis of Lyme borreliosis. In: *International Journal of Medical Microbiology,* (08.08.2011) Available from:
http://www.sciencedirect.com/science?_ob=PublicationURL&_tockey=%23TOC%2320444%232006%23997039999.8998%23622693%23FLA%23&_cdi=20444&_pubType=J&view=c&_auth=y&_acct=C000054081&_version=1&_urlVersion=0&_userid=1647798&md5=bcc5a55f86b9de38d1638add1eaca44a

Kisand, K. E.; Prükk, T. & Kisand, K. V. (2007). Propensity to excessive proinflammatory response in chronic Lyme borreliosis. *Acta Pathologica Microbiologica et Immunologica Scandinavica,* Vol.115, No.2 (February 2007), pp. 134-41, ISSN 1600-0463

Klaska, I. & Nowak, J. Z. (2007). The role of complement in physiology and pathology. *Postępy Higieny i Medycyny Doświadczalnej,*Vol.61, (2007), pp. 167-177, ISSN1732-2693

Krajczy, P.; Skerka, Ch.; Kirschfink, M.; Zipfel, P. F. & Brade, V. (2001). Mechanism of complement resistance of pathogenic Borrelia burgdorferi isolates. *International Immunopharmacology,* Vol.1, No.3, (March 2001), pp. 393-401, ISSN 1567-5769

Liang, F.; Nowling, J. M. & Philipp, M. T. (2000). Cryptic and Expose Invariable Region of VlsE, the Variable Surface Antigen of Borrelia burgdorferi s.l. *Journal of Bacteriology,* Vol.182, No.12, (Jun 2000), pp. 3597-3601, ISSN 1098-5530

Maraspin, V.; Rudzic-Sabljic, E. & Strle, F. (July 2006). Lyme borreliosis and Borrelia spielmani, In: *Emerging Infectious Diseases,* 25.07.2011, Available from:
http://www.cdc.gov/ncidod/EID/vol12no07/06-0077.htm

MMWR (August 1995). Notice to readers recommendations for test performance and interpretation from the Second National Conference on Serologic Diagnosis of Lyme Disease, In: *Center for Disease Control and Prevention,* 14.09.2011, Available from: www.cdc.gov/mmwr/prewiew/mmwrhtml/00038469.htm

Nowak, A. J.; Gilmore, R. D. & Carroll, J. A. (2006). Serologic proteome analysis of Borrelia burgdorferi membrane-associated proteins. *Infection and Immunity*, Vol.74, No.7, (July 2006), pp. 3864 -3873, ISSN 1098-5522

Ołdak, E.; Flisiak, I. & Chodynicka, B. (2009). Lyme borreliosis in children. *Przegląd Dermatologiczny* Vol.96, No. 2, (2009), pp. 146-151, ISSN 0033-2526

Przytuła, L.; Gińdzieńska-Siekiewicz, E. & Sierakowski,S. (2006). Diagnosis and treatment of Lyme arthritis. *Przegląd Epidemiologiczny*, Supl 1, Vol.60, (April 2006), pp. 125-130, PL ISSN 0033-2100

Richter, D.; Schlee, D.B.; Allgower, R. & Matuschka, F. R. (2004). Relationships of a novel Lyme disease spirochete, Borrelia spielmani sp. nov. with its hosts in Central Europe. *Applied Environmental Microbiology*, Vol.70, No.11, (November 2004), pp. 6414-6419, ISSN 1098-5336

Robertson, J.; Guy, E.; Andrews, N.; Wilske, B.; Anda, P.; Granström, M.; Hauser, U.; Moosmann, Y.; Sambri, V.; Schellekens, J.; Stanek, G. & Gray, J. (2000). A European multicenter study of immunobloting in serodiagnosis of Lyme Borreliosis. *Journal of Clinical Microbiology*, Vol.38, No.6, (June 2000), pp. 2097-2102, ISSN: 1098-660X

Ruderko, N.; Golovchenko, M.; Ruzek, D.; Piskunova, N.; Mallátová, N. & Grubhoffer, L. (March 2009). Molecular detection of Borrelia bissettii DNA in serum samples from patients in the Czech Republic with suspected borreliosis, In: *FEMS Microbiology Letters* 25.07.2011, Available from: http://www.ncbi.nlm.nih.gov/pubmed/19187198?ordinalpos=4&itool=EntrezSystem2

Seidel, M. F.; Belda Domene, A.; Vetter, H. (2007). Differential diagnoses of suspected Lyme borreliosis or post-Lyme-disease syndrome. *European Journal of Clinical Microbiology & Infectious Diseases*, Vol.26, No.9, (June 2007), pp.611-617, ISSN 1435-4373

Sicklinger, M.; Winecke, R. & Neubert, U. (2003). In vitro susceptibility testing of four antibiotics against Borrelia burgdorferi: a comparison of results for the three genospecies Borrelia afzelii, Borrelia garinii and Borrelia burgdorferi sensu stricto. *Journal of Clinical Microbiology*, Vol.41, No.4, (April 2003), pp. 1791-1793, ISSN 1098-660X

Siegel, C.; Herzberger, P.; Skerka, Ch.; Brade, V.; Fingerle, V.; Schulze-Spechtel, U.; Wilske, B.; Zipfel, P. F.; Wallich, R. & Kraiczy, P. (1 September 2008). Binding of complement regulatory protein factor H enhances serum resistance of Borrelia spielmani sp. nov. In: *International Journal of Medical Microbiology*, 09.08.2011, Available from: http://www.sciencedirect.com/science/article/pii/S1438422108000052

Siegel, C.; Hallstrom, T.; Skerka, C.; Eberhardt, H.; Uzonyi, B.; Beckhaus, T. & Karas, M. (20 October 2010). Complement factor H-related proteins CFHR2 and CFHR5 represent novel ligands for the infection-associated CRASP proteins of Borrelia burgdorferi, In: *PLoSONE*, 03.08.2011, Available from: http://www.ncbi.nlm.nih.gov/pmc/articles/PMC2958145/?tool=pubmed

Sigal, L. H. (1997). Lyme disease: a review of aspects its immunology and immunopathogenesis. *Annual Reviev of Immunology*, Vol. 15, (April 1997), pp. 63-92, ISSN 0732-0582

Singh, S. K. & Girschick, H. J. (2004a). Molecular survival strategies of the Lyme disease spirochete Borrelia burgdorferi. *The Lancet Infectious Diseases*, Vol.4, No.9 (September 2004), pp. 4575-83, ISSN1473-3099

Singh, S. K. & Girschick, H. J. (2004b). Lyme borreliosis: from infection to autoimmunity. *Clinical Microbiology and Infection*, Vol.10, No.7, (July 2004), pp. 598-614, ISSN 1469-0691

Stanek, G.; Fingerle, V.; Hunfeld, K. P.; Jaulhac, B.; Kaiser, R.; Krause, A.; Kristoferitsch, W.; O'Connell, S.; Ornstein, K.; Strle, F. & Gray, J. (2011). Lyme borreliosis: Clinical case definitions for diagnosis and management in Europe. *Clinical Microbiology and Infection*, Vol.17, No.1, (January 2011), pp. 69-79, ISSN 1469-0691

Štefančiková, A.; Derdáková, M.; Štěpánová, G.; Peťko, B.; Szestáková, E.; Šktardová, I. & Čisláková, L. (2005). Heterogeneity of Borrelia burgdorferi sensu lato and their reflection on immune response. *Annals of Agricultural and Environmental Medicine*, Vol.12, (2005), pp. 211-216, ISSN 1232-1966

Steere, A. C.; Falk, B. & Drobin, E. E. (2003). Binding of outer surface protein A and human lymphocyte function-associated antigen 1 peptides to HLA-DR molecules associated with antibiotic treatment-resistant Lyme arthritis. *Arthritis & Rheumatism*, Vol.48, No.2, (February 2003), pp. 534-40, ISSN 1529-0131

Strasfeld, L.; Romanzi, L.; Seder, R. H. & Berardi, V. (2005). False-positive serological test results for Lyme disease in a patient with acute Herpes Simplex virus type 2 infection. *Clinical Infectious Diseases*, Vol.41, No.12, (December 2005), pp. 1826-1827 1537-6591

Suchonen, J.; Hartiala, K.; Tuominen-Gusstafson, H. & Viljanen, M. K. Sublethal concentrations of complement can effectively opsonize Borrelia burgdorferi. (2002). *Scandinavian Journal of Immunology*, Vol.56, No.6, (December 2002), pp. 554-560, ISSN 1365-3083

Suhonen, J.; Hartiala, K.; Tuominen-Gustafsson, H. & Viljanen, M. K. (2000). Borrelia burgdorferi - induced oxidative burst, calcium mobilization and phagocytosis of human neutrophils are complement dependent. *The Journal of Infectious Diseases*, Vol.181, No.1, (January 2000), pp. 195-202, ISSN 0022-1899

Śpiewak, R.; Stojek, N. M. & Chmielewska-Badora, J.(2004). Antinuclear antibodies are not increased in the early phase of Borrelia infection. *Annals of Agricultural and Environmental Medicine*, Vol.11, (2004), pp. 145-148, ISSN 1232-1966

Tokarska-Rodak, M.; Fota-Markowska, H.; Śmiechowicz, F.; Gajownik, B.; Prokop, M.; Modrzewska, R. & Kozioł-Montewka, M. (2010a). Antibodies against in vivo B. burgdorferi antigens evaluated in patients with Lyme arthritis with reference to treatment. *Advances in Clinical and Experimental Medicine*, Vol.19, No.4, (2010). pp. 489-496, ISSN1230-025X

Tokarska-Rodak, M.; Niedźwiadek, J.; Fota-Markowska, H.; Śmiechowicz, F.; Gajownik, B.; Modrzewska, R. & Kozioł-Montewka, M. (2010b). Antinuclear antibodies in patients with Lyme disease. *New Medicine*, Vol.XIV, No.4, (2010), pp. 152-155, ISSN 1427-0994

Tokarska-Rodak, M; Fota-Markowska, H.; Kozioł-Montewka, M; Śmiechowicz, F. & Modrzewska, R. (2010c). The detection of specific antibodies against B. burgdorferi s.s., B. afzelii, B. garinii and B. spielmani antigens in patients with Lyme disease in the Eastern Poland. *New Medicine*, Vol.XIV, No.3, (2010), pp. 84-87, ISSN 1427-0994

Tokarska-Rodak, M.; Kozioł-Montewka, M.; Fota-Markowska, H.; Bielec, D.; Modrzewska, R. & Pańczuk, A. (2008). Frequency and specificity of the antibodies against Borrelia burgdorferi tested by Western blot method in patients with symptoms of arthritis. *Central European Journal of Immunology*, Vol.33, No.4, (2008), pp. 220-223, ISSN 1426-3912

Tokarska-Rodak, M.; Kozioł-Montewka, M.; Pańczuk, A.; Fota-Markowska, H. & Modrzewska, R. (2007). Borelioza z Lyme-problemy diagnostyczne i rehabilitacyjne, In: *Problemy osób niepełnosprawnych,* Turowski Krzysztof, Paluszkiewicz Piotr, Spisacka Stanisława, pp. 33-36,WSZ, ISBN 978-83-923366-7-9, Biała Podlaska

Wang, G.; Van Dam, A. P. & Dankert, J. (1999). Phenotypic and genetic characterization of a novel Borrelia burgdorferi sensu lato isolate from a patient with Lyme borreliosis. *Journal of Clinical Microbiology* Vol.37, No.9, (September 1999), pp. 3025-3028, ISSN 1098-660X

Wilgat, P.; Pancewicz, S.; Hermanowska-Szpakowicz, T.; Kondrusik, M.; Zajkowska, J.; Grygorczuk. S.; Popko, J. & Zwierz, K. (2004). Activity of lisosomal exoglycosidases in serum of patients with chronic borrelia arthritis. *Przegląd Epidemiologiczny,* Vol.58, No.3, (2004), pp. 451-458, ISSN 0033-2100

Wilske, B. (2003). Diagnosis of Lyme borreliosis in Europe. *Victor-Borne and Zoonotic Diseases.* Vol.3, No.4 (2003). pp. 215-227, ISSN 1557-7759

Wilske, B.; Fingerle, V. & Schulte-Spechtel, U. (2007). Microbiological and serological diagnosis of Lyme borreliosis. *FEMS Immunology & Medical Microbiology* Vol.49, No.1, (February 2007), pp. 13-21, ISSN 1574-695X

Wodecka, B. (2006a). Borrelia burgdorferi - charakterystyka ewolucyjna i molekularna, In: *Biologia molekularna patogenów przenoszonych przez kleszcze,* Stokarczyk Bogumiła, pp. 97. Wydawnictwo Lekarskie PZWL, ISBN-10: 83-200-3490-6, Warszawa

Wodecka, B (2006b). Metody diagnostyczne polecane w boreliozie z Lyme, In: *Biologia molekularna patogenów przenoszonych przez kleszcze,* Stokarczyk Bogumiła, pp. 142 Wydawnictwo Lekarskie PZWL, ISBN-10: 83-200-3490-6, Warszawa

Zajkowska, J.; Kondrusik, M.; Pancewicz, S.; Grygorczuk, S.; Wierzbińska, R.; Hermanowska-Szpakowicz, T.; Czeczuga, A. & Sienkiewicz, I. (2006a). Western-Blot with VlsE protein and „in vivo" antigens in Lyme borreliosis diagnosis. *Przegląd Epidemiologiczny,* Vol.60, Supl 1, (April 2006), pp.177-185, ISSN 0033-2100

Zajkowska, J.; Kondrusik, M.; Pancewicz, S.A.; Sienkiewicz, I.; Grygorczuk, S.; Wierzbińska, R. & Hermanowska-Szpakowicz, T. (2006b). Laboratory diagnosis of early Lyme borreliosis-comparison of ELISA, Western blot (EcoLine), and PCR results. *International Journal of Medical Microbiology,* Vol.296, No.S1, (2006), pp. 291-293, ISSN 1438-4221

Zajkowska, J.; Grygorczuk, S.; Kondrusik, M.; Pancewicz, S. & Hermanowska-Szpakowicz, T. (2006c). New aspects of pathogenesis of Lyme borreliosis. *Przegląd Epidemiologiczny,* Vol.60, Supl 1 (April 2006), pp. 167-170, ISSN 0033-210

5

Discovering Lyme Disease in Ticks and Dogs in Serbia – Detection and Diagnostic Methods

Sara Savic
DVM, Scientific Veterinary Institute „Novi Sad", Novi Sad
Serbia

1. Introduction

Lyme disease is one of the infectious diseases discovered in the last three decades. It is a systemic, infectious and zooantropoic disease. Lyme disease is caused by spirochetes *Borrelia burgdorferi* s.l., and is primarily transferred via *Ixodes* ticks. Ticks that are vectors for Lyme disease in Europe and also in Serbia are from *Ixodes ricinus* species (Burgdorfer et all, 1989). Up to date the existence of 13 strains of *Borreliae burgdoerferi sensu lato*, is confirmed and only three of them are pathogens for humans and animals: *B. burgdorferi sensu stricto, B. afzelii* and *B. garinii*. After natural infections of dogs with pathogen strains of *B. burgdorferi* s.l. clinical symptoms are found in 5% of infected dogs. In most of the cases clinical symptoms are similar to a second stadium of Lyme disease in humans - anorexia, weakness, lymphadenopathia, increase of body temperature. Later, 2-5 months after a tick bite an intermittent lameness can be found.

There are no characteristic clinical symptoms and that makes diagnostic of Lyme disease quite a challenge. That is why laboratory diagnostic is necessary and sometimes the only way to correct diagnosis. Laboratory diagnostic is based on detection of specific antibodies against *B. burgdorferi* s.l. in blood serum and synovial fluid; isolation and detection of *B. burgdorferi* s.l. genome with molecular method.

During the last five years a certain percentage of ticks infected with *B. burgorferi* s.l. has been discovered (25 - 30% in different regions) in Serbia (Milutinović et al 2008, Cekanac et all 2009). Also, clinical cases of the disease are found in dogs and humans.

2. History

Lyme disease is actually present in many countries and only in Europe; over 19 countries have confirmed the existence of the disease (Burgdorfer, 1991). According to the literature data, several studies have been done in the country and in the surrounding countries in the domain of veterinary and human medicine on Lyme disease and on tick infections with *B.burgdorferi*. The first human case of Lyme borreliosis in USA was detected in 1975. From that time, numerous studies have been done in different countries and regions (Duncan et all, 2005). Prevalence for Lyme disease found in dogs in Alabama and North Carolina was rather low, even under 3%, while in New Jersey the prevalence was over 30% and in Wiskonsin, New York and Connecticut it was over 50% (Magnarelli et all 1988, Shulze et all 1987, Wright et all

1997). Since 1995. Until today, human cases of Lyme disease have been reported in 48 countries in USA. Sudies done in Europe have shown various data. In northwestern part of Croatia 45% of ticks were infected with *B.burgdorferi s.l.* (Golubić et all, 1998). In Lublin region,Poland, over 60% of ticks infected with causative agent of Lyme disease were found (Cisak et all, 2006.). Data for Switzerland, implicate that 19% of ticks were infected with *B.burgdorferi s.l.* (Moran Cadenas et all, 2007). In Portugal, during the past 15 years, cases of Lyme disease in humans were reported in 17 regions, from 20 regions in total, while prevalence in ticks was found from 11/35% (Lopes de Carvalho and Nuncio, 2006.). Research done in Spain resulted in similar data for prevalence of 11% in dogs and humans (Merino et all, 2000.), even though *I.ricinus* is not dominant population of ticks - only 12% of total tick population are *I.ricinus* ticks(Merino et all, 2005.). After the research was done in Check Republoc, 30% of ticks were found to be infected with B.burgdorferi s.l. (Hulinska et all 2007.).

In Serbia some research is done in the region of Belgrade, where 20-30% of ticks are infected with *B.burgdorferi,* in 2004, seroprevalence in ticks was 21,8 %(Milutinović et all, 2004; Čekanac et all, 2009) and in 2005, it was 17,5%. During a few years period (2001-2004) infection was found to be even 42% in the selected sample of ticks (Milutinović et all, 2008). In Resavica region, during 2007, infection of ticks was on average 33,6%. In Vojvodina region (northern part of Serbia), during a period from 2004-2007, 22-28% of infected ticks were found (Jurišić, 2005; Savić-Jevđenić et all, 2007). In Belgrade (capital of Serbia) Lyme disease was detected in 1987, for the first time (Dmitrović, Popović, 1993; Lako et all, 1998), and later on in the other parts of Serbia. In the autumn of 1989 in a daily newspaper an announcement from Prof. dr Boriša Vuković (at that time a Director of Epidemiology service, Medical faculty Novi Sad) was published: "If there was not AIDS, Lyme disease would surely be No 1 disease in its spreading and epidemiological value, among the new disease". Since December 1989, Lyme disease is obligatory for announcing if appears, in Serbia. From 1991 to 2004, 7774 people are registered for having Lyme disease. Of all those patients, 47,8% were from the territory of Belgrade and 23,7% of the patients were from Vojvodina region. Incidence for Vojvodina was from 0,4 in 1991, to 11,7 in 2004 (Epidemiological bulletin, 2005).

According to the data from Medical Clinical Center of Vojvodina, number of humans that had clinical symptoms of Lyme disease with laboratory conformation of diagnosis during the last 5 years was the following:

- 2006 28 patients;
- 2007 48 patients;
- 2008 54 patients;
- 2009 40 patients;
- 2010 53 patients;
- 2011 33 patients in the first 8 months;

In 2008, there were 50% more patients then in 2006 and then in the following period the annual number of patients was more or less the same. According to the report in Health and statistical yearbook of Serbia published by Institut for public health of Serbia „Dr Milan Jovanović Batut", the number of patients with Lyme disease in Serbia was in total 651 during 2007, of wich 456 were in central Serbia and 195 cases were in Vojvodina. Lyme disease cases make 97% of all vector borne diseases recorded in 2007 in Serbia and 99% in Vojvodina.

3. Ecology, epidemiology – life cycle of ticks and tranfer of the causative agent

The best conditions for tick's life cycle in Serbia can be found in the regions between woods and meadows and also between deciduous and evergreen forests. Geographical position of the localities, elevation, composition of flora and fauna, presence of the hosts, vectors and enough food for rodents represent the optimal conditions for maintenance and circulation of *B.burgdorferi* s.l. The most important factor that influences the quality of tick's life is air humidity. In mixed woods, the tick population is highest in the places where humidity reaches 70-80%. Little paths through woods, which are used by forest animals, are the places with a highest risk for humans and animals.

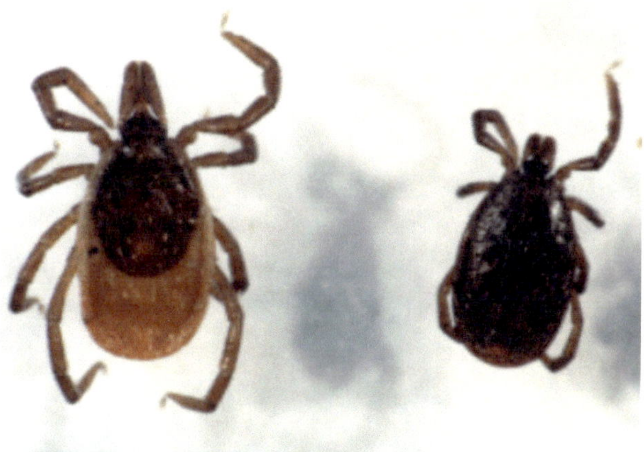

Picture 1. *I. ricinus*, adults female and male, Jurišić (2008)

Ticks, infected and not infected can often be found in urban parks with woods, very near to the big cities. Appearance of ticks in the cities seems to be connected to development of new parks and woods and also building of urban parts on the edge of a forest. The survival of ticks in certain localities is determined by a possibility to realize the whole life cycle of ticks with all the hosts needed and developing stages (Wall, Shearer, 1992; Pejchalova, 2007).

A dominant species of ticks that carry Lyme disease in Serbia is *Ixodes ricinus*. This tick has a two season phase in life cycle - spring and autumn phase. During the tick season, a change in prevalence of Lyme disease can be expected. Research done during the '90-ties, when *B. burgdorferi* s.l. was isolated for the first time in the region of Belgrade, until nowadays show that infection of ticks with *B. burgdorferi* s.l. is from 20-30%, with a mild trend of growth (Milutinović et all, 2004). For the region of Vojvodina, this percentage is from 25-28% (Jurišić, 2005; 2008; Savić -Jevđenić et all, 2007).

On the localities in the urban parts, ticks were mostly found in woods and parks with woods and the smallest number of ticks was found in landscaped parks, because the treatment against ticks was always performed there, during the spring period. Besides that, in woods and parks with woods the influence of mankind is less, so these places are rich in flora and fauna, compared to the localities in urban places. Based on the research done during the period from 2002-2004, author Jurišić concludes that far most common tick species, present in urban regions is *Ixodes ricinus* (Jurišić, 2005). Depending on the weather conditions, the presence of ticks was spotted until the beginning of October, in 2003, and in 2004 the tick activity was registered during the whole year, with the maximal periods - the last one in November when air temperatures were below 8°C and relative air humidity over 85%. During this three year period, infection of ticks was analyzed in chosen localities of urban regions. In total 461 ticks from different locations was analyzed for the presence of *B. burgdorferi* s.l. spirochetes and mean infection of 25% in ticks was determined. In several chosen localities where no chemical treatment was ever used, the infection of ticks reached 29% and the lowest infection rate of 16% was determined in the urban parts of cities (Jurišić 2005; Jurišić, 2008).

Lindgren and Jaenson, while working on project about the influence of climate changes to the presence of Lyme disease, concluded that from the '80-ties, density and spreading of ticks has increased towards higher latitude and longitude. The climate changes announced for Europe will bring to spreading of Lyme disease to higher latitude and longitude. On the other hand in some regions where Lyme disease can be found now, when climate becomes too hot and dry for tick survival, Lyme disease might disappear from those regions. According to the prediction in the next 50 years, the climate in Europe will become milder, with higher winter air temperatures and longer vegetation period with higher risk of floods in the north of Europe and dry air in the southern parts of Europe. All of these elements can influence directly the number and distribution of ticks and their hosts in the region (Lindgren and Jaenson, 2004).

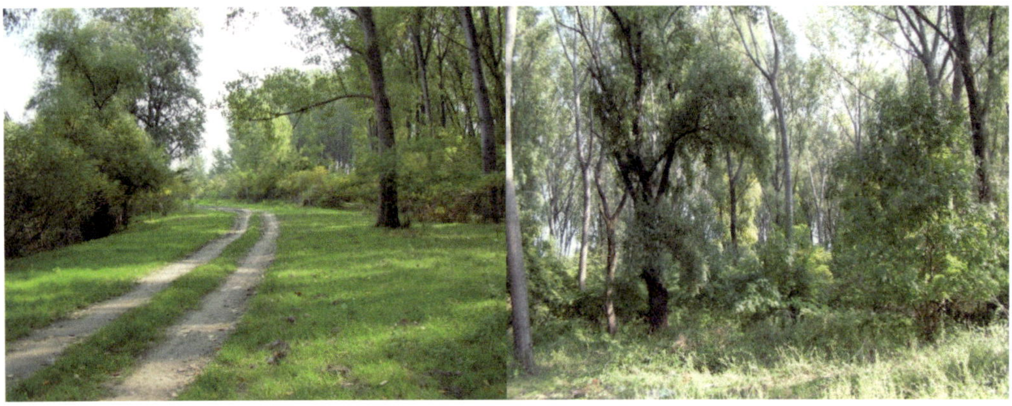

Pictures 2. and 3. -Woods near the urban region where infected ticks were found.

3.1 Pathogenesis and immunological response

Criteria for clinical diagnostic of Lyme disease in dogs are defined in 1992: anorexia, depression, malfunction of limbs or joints. After a natural infection clinical symptoms may appear even few months after the infection as lameness and joint swelling, which lasts for 3-4 days and then the symptoms may disappear and then reappear after a few weeks or months (Epidemiological bulletin, 2005). A research was done on hound dogs aiming to highlight that weather there are dogs without any clinical symptoms or those with typical clinical symptoms, total prevalence for Lyme borreliosis is 15-20% (Savić-Jevđenić et all, 2008).

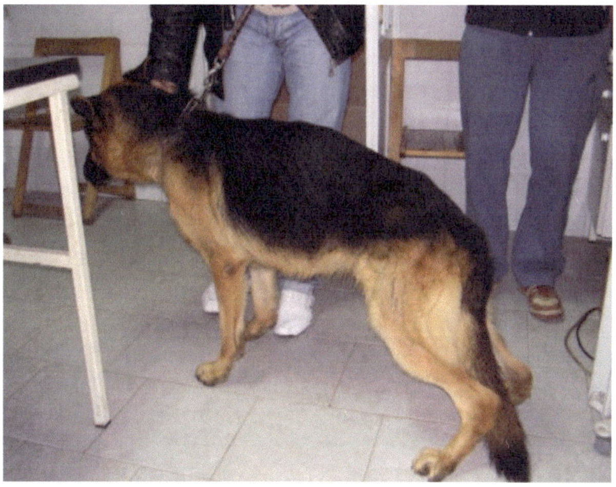

Picture 4. German shepherd with lameness and positive serological finding for Lyme disease (Veterinary practice „Leo", Novi Sad, Lolić, 2008.)

In dogs there is no erythema migrans stage, but there can be skin leisure after tick bite. After natural infection with *B.burgdorferi* a renal malfunction can appear in form of glomerulonephritis and changes in renal tubule, but renal malfunction are not characteristic only for Lyme boreliosis. There are no changes in hematological and biochemical blood parameters in cases of Lyme disease (Dmitrović and Popović, 1993).

4. Diagnostic

Diagnostic of borreliosis is based on epidemiology, epizootiology, clinical symptoms, laboratory tests and reaction to antibiotic treatment (Skotarczak, 2007). Standard serology tests are based on detection of specific antibodies produced in dog's organism against *B. burgdoerferi* s.l. Many animals get into contact with *B. burgdorferi* s.l. and consequently antibodies appear, but there are no clinical symptoms. In Serbia there is no regular vaccination against Lyme borreliosis. Dogs suspicious for Lyme boreliosis have to have a history of tick bite, some clinical symptoms and a good response to antibiotic treatment and those are four important criteria in diagnostic of Lyme borreliosis (Dmitrović and Popović 1993). Laboratory testing has to be validated in order to be useful in diagnostic of Lyme disease because false positive and false negative findings are possible (Jacobson et all, 1996). According to the OIE Manual, recommended methods for diagnostic of Lyme disease are ELISA test, indirect fluorescence (IFA) or immunoblot method (Western blot). Dogs disposed to *B.burgdorferi* s.l. are in 95% cases seropositive, but asymptomatic carriers of the disease.

4.1 Field research

Field research was done by field collecting of ticks with „flag" method. Chosen localities for tick collecting were in Northern part of Serbia, province of Vojvodina and localities in Fruska Gora mountain. Localities were chosen with different vegetation, from simple grass fields, fields with weeds by the channel and river with sandy soil, to forested sites of Fruska Gora mountain - urban sites, parks, abounded settlements, suburbs, green fileds and settlements beside Danube river, forestery sites in Fruska Gora, enbankments. The conditions and habitats were optimal for tick life cycle. Also animals and humans were present in the chosen localities and sites. Localities were chosen according to the previeus history of tick bites in humans and dogs, previous research on tick infection with *B. burgdorferi* s.l. and seroprevelance in dogs for Lyme disease. Ticks were collected from the end of March to the beginning of June and then again from August until the end of October. From all the ticks collected, after identification, only *Ixodes ricinus* ticks were further analyzed. Pools were made on the basis of stage and gender and by microscopy in dark field ticks abdomen was explored and analyzed for the presence of spirochetes. When spirochetes were found, the samples of the abdomen content were inoculated into liquid BSK-H complete medium (Sigma medium complete with 6% of rabbit serum) and kept at 33°C (Cisak et all, 2006; Pejchelova, 2007). Examination of ticks was done according to the work of Milutinović et all, 2004.

During a three year period, 1224 ticks were collected from different localities and 62% of them were *Ixodes ricinus.* After examination of tick abdomen, the annual percentage of infected ticks is shown in Table 1. There is an uphill trend of infected ticks during the three year period. *I. ricinus* ticks were 60-64% (764) of the total number of ticks during the research period and 22,12% of those ticks were infected with *B. burgdorferi* s.l. During the research in 2008, in one region none of the ticks were infected with *B. burgdorferi s.l.*, and in one urban region with surroundings, infected ticks were 29,2%.

Year	No of collected ticks	% I. ricinus	No and % of adult females	No and % of adult males	No and % of nymphs	**No and % of ticks infected with B.b.**
2006.	386	232 (60%)	109 (47%)	102 (44%)	21(9%)	**44 (18,9%)**
2007.	479	302 (63%)	173 (57%)	93 (31%)	36(12%)	**94 (19,6%)**
2008.	359	230 (64%)	90 (39%)	119 (52%)	21(9%)	**55 (23,8%)**
TOTAL	**1224**	**764 (62%)**	**372 (49%)**	**314 (41%)**	**78(10%)**	**169(22,12%)**

Table 1. Number of examined and infected *I.ricinus* ticks for the presence of *B.burgdorfer* s.l.i, in period 2006 - 2008.

4.2 Entomological Risk Index (ERI)

By defining ERI, the possibility of Lyme disease risk estimation for human population in a certain region can be defined. Mather et all used standard protocols to define density of tick population and their infection in different localities. Authors have also stated a positive correlation between ERI and number of Lyme disease cases in certain localities, meaning that a risk from Lyme disease for a certain region can be predicted by calculating ERI (Mather et all 1996). ERI for a certain period of research is calculated as number of collected ticks in one minute multiplied by the tick infection level. For the regions where ticks were collected, ERI was calculated in relation to a total number of collected ticks (shown in Table 2).

Region	No of collected ticks in hour	No of collected ticks in minute (NT)	Level of tick infection (TI)	ERI
Settlements Region	4	0,067	0,234	0,016
Region of FruskaGora woods	6	0,100	0,290	0,029
Urban region with surroundings	11	0,183	0,292	0,053
Mean value	**7,3**	**0,122**	**0,272**	**0,033**

Table 2. No of ticks collected in one minute (NT), level of tick infection (TI) and ERI values in the studied regions

The greatest ERI was found in urban region, because the biggest level of tick infection and total number of collected ticks was also found in the same region.

4.3 Laboratory analysis

4.3.1 Isolation and cultivation of *Borrelia burgdorferi spp*

Isolation was done on selective mediom BSK-H complete medium, Sigma, according to Current Protocols in Mycrobiology (Zuckert, 2007, Pejchelova 2007). Tubes with medium and inoculated material were kept at 33-34°C and after the growing of spirochetes was noticed they were recultured into a new tube, under microaerophilic conditions for growing. Typisation of spirochetes was done by a molecular method. From 26 pools cultured in total, in 4 of them (15%) the growth of spirochetes was observed and they were named after the localities they were collected at:

1. „Granicar 1" (pool 1, 5 male adult ticks from a non settled locality);
2. „Granicar 2" (pool 2, 5 adult male ticks from a non settled locality);
3. „244" (pool of 5 adult female ticks from a settled locality);
4. „Novi Sad" (pool of 5 adult ticks from the urban locality).

In first, second and third pool, growth of spirochetes was noticed after 14 days and in fourth pool after 21 days. Concentration of gained isolates of *B. burgdoerferi spp* was the following:

1. „Granicar 1" : 32 X 10^5 *B. burgdorferi* / ml of culture;
2. „Granicar 2" : 32 X 10^5 *B. burgdorferi* / ml of culture ;
3. „244" : 72 X 10^5 *B. burgdorferi* / ml of culture;
4. „Novi Sad" : 76 X 10^5 *B. burgdorferi* / ml of culture.

Detection of specific antibodies against *B. burgdorferi s.l.* was done with serologic methods CF, ELISA, Western blot and fast test. The observation for the apperiance of clinical symptoms of Lyme disease was also done. In the localities where ticks were collected, blood sampling from dogs was done, for serological survey. Dogs blood samples are deviden into three groups by their usage, region and existing clinical symptoms of Lyme disease.

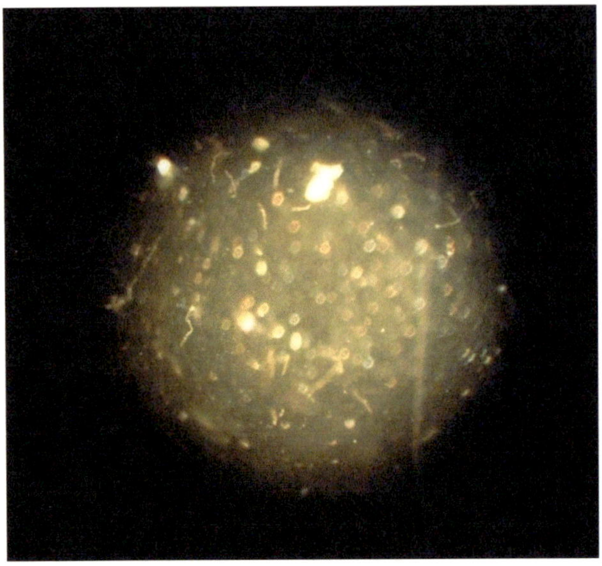

Picture 5. Spirochetes of „Novi Sad" isolate in dark field

5. Serology

Serology was done in the blood serum from dogs naturaly infected *B. burgdorferi* s.l. Samples were from:

- dogs with clinical symptoms of Lyme disease,
- dogs pets without any clinical symptoms, from the region where *B. burgdorferi* s.l. was found to be present in ticks,
- hunting dogs and military dogs without any clinical symptoms, from the region where *B. burgdorferi* s.l. was found to be present in ticks.

CF (complement fixation) method was done in microtitar plates, using produsers instructions of Virion (*B. burgdorferi* s.l. antigen). Samples were diluted until 1:10 in veronal puffer and general principles of CF method were used with 2% erythrocytes in Elsevier's solution.

Method ELISA is performed by using the kis for detection of specific antibodies against *B. burgdorferi* s.l. by Mikrogen, Germany - recomWell Borrelia canis IgG and recomWell Borrelia canis IgM. This enzyme immunotest contains recombinant antigens for the detection of IgG or IgM antibodies against *B. burgdorferi sensu stricto, B. garinii and B. afzelii*, in dog's serum or plasma samples. This is a quantitative test for detection and identification of IgG or IgM antibodies and represents a screening test based on the principles of indirect sandwich ELISA. By using recombinant proteins, the usage of protein combinations of different *B. burgdorferi* genospecies in one test is possible and by selecting specific antigens, important for a sensitive serologic diagnostic, the influence of cross reactions in the test is very low. In this ELISA test, proteins of the outer membrane OspC and specific inner part of p41 antigen (flagelin) are used and also a very specific *B. burgdorferi* s.l. antigens like p100, VisE and p18 (a bounding protein A, Osp17). Although, it is possible that if the analysis is done in the real early phase of infection when there are not enough antibodies yet, that a false negative finding appears. Therapy with antibiotics in the early stage of the disease can also reduce the amount of antigens needed and that way influence the results of ELISA test. So, the producer recommends that if the ELISA findings are negative and clinical symptoms exist, a new sample and testing should be done after three weeks. False positive results are also possible, because antibodies persist in the organism for a long time and they can be from a previous old infection, still high enough to induce a positive finding. That is why it is recommended to confirm a positive finding by another method, like Western blot. The findings after ELISA test have o be interpreted together with having in mind clinical symptoms.

Western blott test is performed by using the kits according to the producers instructions Mikrogen for diagnostic kit recomBlot Borrelia Canis IgG. RecomBlot Borrelia canis is a qualitative test for in vitro detection and assured identification of IgG or IgM antibodies against *B. burgdorferi* s.l. in serum or plasma from dogs. This test can be used for verification of the results gained after a screening test. In recomBlot Borrelia canis test, specific *B.burgdorferi* s.l. antigens are used which are produced with recombinant cells of *E. colli.* Antigens used in the reaction are proteins of outer surface OspA and OspC, and also highly specific B. *burgdorferi* antigens p100, p39 and p18, and also p41 (flagelin). In recomBlot Borrelia canis test OspC protein from all three genospecies can be found. By immuno blot testing it is possible to distinguish a natural infection from vaccination. A negative finding still does not completely rule out the possibility of *B. burgdorferi* s.l. infection, especially in the very early phase of infection, when there are still not enough antibodies produced in the organism. Also, antibiotic treatment in the really early stage of infection can prevent forming detectible antibodies. If there are clinical symptoms for Lyme disease and a negative finding by Western blot method, the reaction should be repeated three weeks later. In the early stage of infection, IgM antibodies are predominant and reaction with OspC and p41 (IgM). In the later stage of infection, beside with OspC and p41, there is a strong reaction also with p100 and VisE. Detection of IgG antibodies against p100, p39 or p18 is enough for a positive finding.

A fast test FASTest Lyme, by Mega Cor Diagnostik, Austria is a sensitive and reliable method, based on specific imunochromatography. It is produced so that IgG and IgM antibodies can be detected in dog's blood serum or plasma. In the test there is a unique combination of specifically marked antigens, with conjugate color. For performing the test there are no special conditions needed and the result comes out in 15 minutes. In endemic regions a seropositive finding can be gained, without any clinical symptoms, so every positive result has to be confirmed by a specific ELISA or Western blot test.

Blood samples from dogs were divided into three groups:

In the first group there were 145 blood samples from working and hunting dogs that live in the regions where ticks were collected previously. All the dogs in this group were regularly vaccinated and treated against ecto and endo parasites, age from 1 to 10, or different breeds - Hungarian visla, German hunting terrier, Labrador, pullin, Rottweiler, epaniel Breton, German Sheppard and sarplaninac . These dogs were constantly exposed to ticks, every day and in 19 (13%) dogs the ticks were found while blood sampling. In 64 (44%) dogs at least one tick was found in the previous period. These dogs are used for hunting, field work or military purposes. With CF test a positive finding was gained in 22,1% of samples. In the samples from the region where infected ticks were not found, there were also no positive finding by serology, with CF and ELISA. The greatest number of dogs with positive serology findings for specific antibodies against *B. burgdorferi s.l.* was in the region of settlements 37,9% by CF and 34,5% by ELISA test. In total, the percentage of dogs from firs group that have specific antibodies against *B. burgdorferi s.l.* is 22,1% by CF method, 22,4 % by ELISA test and 18% by Western blot method.

In the second group there were 16 blood samples from dogs with clinical symptoms interpreted as Lyme disease symptoms - lameness, difficult waking, repeated lameness in different limbs, loss of appetite, occasional elevation of body temperature 39,5-40°C, weakness, with a history of tick bite in the last 2 months. In dogs from this group clinical symptoms were observed. This was done with a help of veterinary practices from the region. Six of these dogs were on a nonspecific unsuccessful treatment with antibiotics of wide range before the blood analysis. These dogs had a repetition of lameness every time the antibiotic treatment was stopped. The serology tests done in these dogs were fast test, CF, ELISA and Western blott. As a result a positive serological finding was gained in 15 dogs by CF, in 14 dogs by ELISA and Western blott and in 13 dogs by fast test. In two dogs specific antibodies against B. *burgdorferi* s.l. were not found by four serology tests. In the same 13 samples the presence of specific antibodies against *B. burgdorferi* s.l., were found with four different serology tests.

In the third group there were 486 blood samples from dogs which were brought for different analysis (piroplasmosis, leptspirosis, leishmaniosis, noninfective digestive malfunctions, urinary problems, ascites, bacterial skin infections, dirofilariosis, respiratory problems, etc), with clinical symptoms not related to Lyme disease. These dogs were kept as pets, mostly in the urban region with surrounding and some from the Fruska Gora Mountain. Dogs were from 2-14 years old. In this group were also samples from 39 dogs living in two dog shelters, all dogs were older than 5 years with an "unknown history". All of these dogs came from the region where ticks were collected previously and where ticks infected with *B. burgdorferi* s.l. were found (29%). Serology was done by CF method, and then positive samples were tested with ELISA and Western blot method. By CF method a positive finding was gained in 32,9% of samples (24,3% in dilution 1:10 and 8,6% in dilution 1:20). By ELISA test a positive finding was gained for IgM antibodies in 19,3% of samples and for IgG in 25,5% of samples. In total, positive serology finding by ELISA was gained in 29,6% of blood samples from the dogs in the third group. By Western blott positive serology finding was gained in 26,1%. In 107 samples analyzed (out of 127 with positive finding) a p100 was detected, which is characteristic for *B. afzelii*. In 55 samples protein BmpA (39) was detected, also characteristic for *B. afzelii*, and in 54 samples VisE was found, which is characteristic for different genospecies. In 22 samples protein p41 was found, characteristic for *B. burgdorferi* sensu stricto. OspA characteristic for *B. afzelii* were detected in 18 samples and OspC characteristic for different genospecies were detected in 19 samples. The highest number of samples gave positive findings for the proteins characteristic for *B. afzelii*.

A comparative display of the findings after serology test of three groups of dogs blood serums analyzed for the presence of specific antibodies against *B. burgdorferi* s.l. by four serology methods - fast test, CF, ELISA and Western blot is given in Table 3. The highest number of positive findings was gained by CF method (32%), then by ELISA (29,91%) and by Western blot (25,81%). In the total of 631 dogs blood samples without clinical symptoms of Lyme disease living in the region where seroprevalence in ticks is 22%, a seroprevalence for Lyme disease in dogs was found to be 21,4% - 32,9%, depending on the method used.

No of group	Total No of samples	No of positive samples to B.b.s.l. by fast test	No of positive samples to B.b.s.l. by CF	No of positive samples to B.b.s.l. by ELISA IgM	No of positive samples to B.b.s.l. by ELISA IgG	No of positive samples to B.b.s.l. by ELISA	No of pos. samp.to B.b.s.l. W.blott
I	145	-	32 (22,1%)	15 (10,3%)	27 (18,6%)	31* (21,4%)	26 (18%)
II	16	13 (81,25%)	15 (93,75%)	3 (18,7%)	11 (68,7%)	14* (87,5%)	14 (87,5%)
III	486	-	160 (32,9%)	94 (19,3%)	124 (25,5%)	144* (29,6%)	127 (26,1%)
Total	647	13	207 (32%)	112 (17,31%)	162 (25,04%)	189* (29,91%)	167 (25,81%)

Not a simple adding of positive IgG and IgM, because of overlapping in some samples of positive finding to IgG and IgM ELISA (74 samples in total)

Table 3. Results of analysed blood samples from dogs, for the presence of specific antibodies against *B. burgdorferi* s.l.with four serology tests

6. Molecular analysis

PCR (Polymerasa Chain Reaction) and Real Time-PCR were used for identification of *B. burgdorferi* s.l. isolated from ticks and typisation of genospecies from isolates of *B. burgdorferi* s.l. from ticks. Isolation of total DNA was done with QIAamp® DNA Mini kit, with „spin-column" procedure of „QIAGEN", Germany. Identification of *B. burgdorferi* was done by real time PCR method with a diagnostic kit PCRFast® *Borrelia burgdorferi* Realtime (SYBR®Green) and / or gel detection, Germany. In case of realtime (SYBR®Green) positive findings, a verification has to be done by analysis od dissosiation curve and evaluation of exponential curve of amplification. For that purpose the picks of dissosiation curve belonging to the sample are compared with the ones belonging to the inhibition control ITC. In estimation of the results exponential curve of amplificatin and dissosiation curve are beeing analysed. Exponential curve of amplification of the sample and inhibition control ITC are beeing compared and they should have similar values. In positive samples dissosiation curve and curve of inhibition control should be at the same level. In negative samples there is no dissociation curve or it is different from the dissociation curve of inhibiton control ITC (Picture 6).

Dissociation curves from samples of isolated cultures from field ticks had similar values with dissociation curve for each positive control, inhibition control ITC, meaning that the samples were positive for the presence of *B. burgdorferi* s.l. DNA. *B. burgdorferi* s.l. is identified in the cultures of spirochetes isolated from field ticks. For the isolate „Novi Sad" pick temperature of dissociation curve was 79,0°C, and pick temperature of ITC for the same sample was 79,4°C.

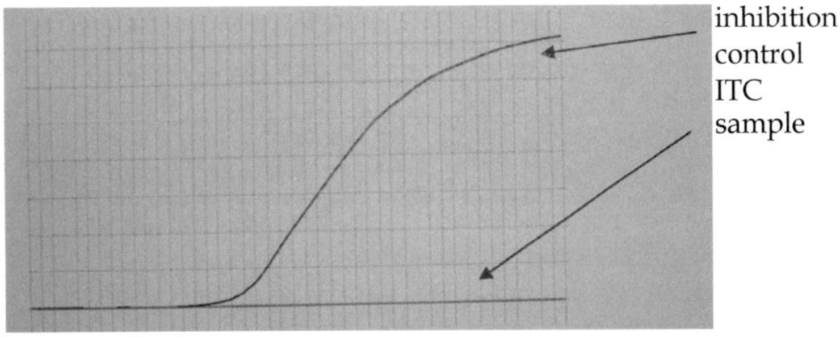

Negative sample

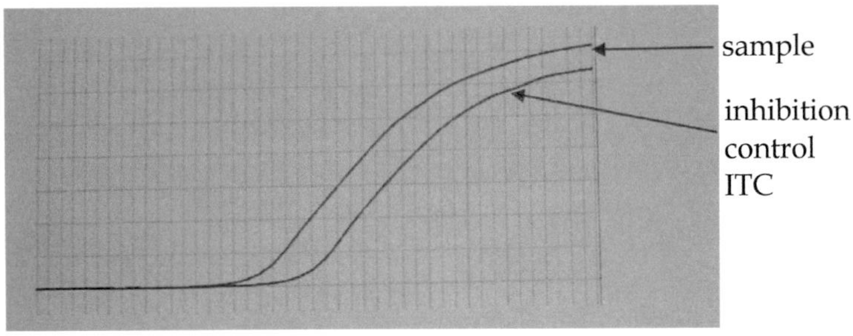

Positive sample

Picture 6. Evaluation of dissosiation curve

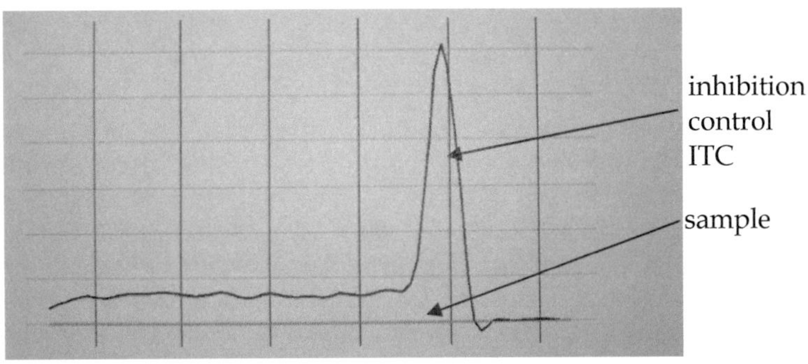

Negative sample

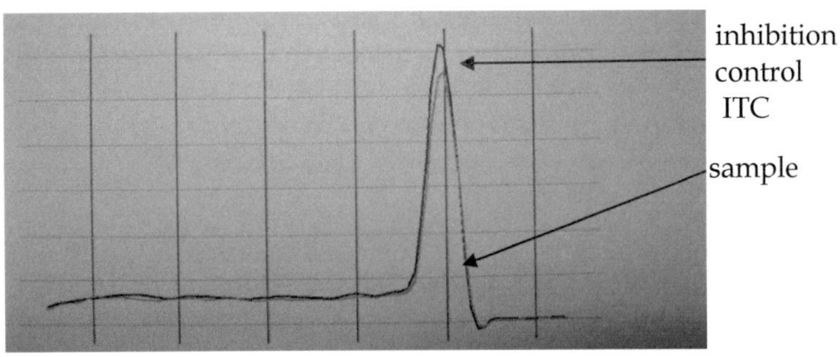

Positive sample

Picture 7. Evaluation of exponential curve of amplification

Typisation of *B. burgdorferi* s.l. isolates from ticks was done by PCR technique and the results were the following:

1. „Granicar 1" : *Borrelia afzelii* (specific fragment 591bp);
2. „Granicar 2" : *Borrelia afzelii* (specific fragment 591bp);
3. „244" : *B. burgdorferi sensu stricto* (specific fragment 575bp);
4. „Novi Sad" : *Borrelia afzelii* (specific fragment 591bp).

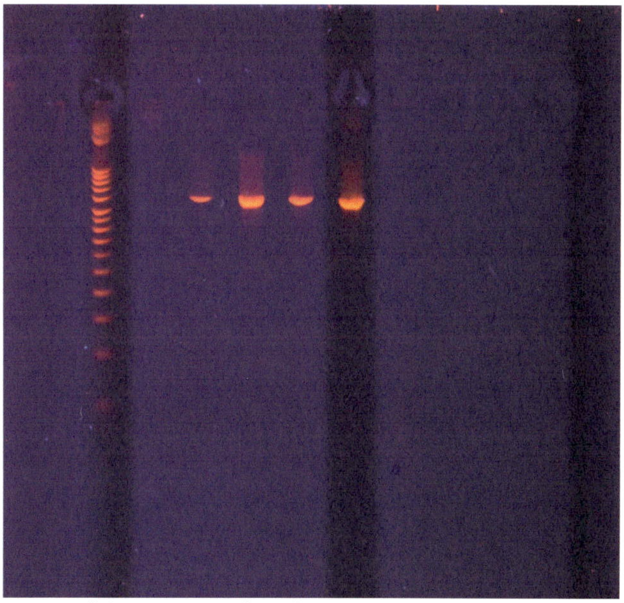

M 1 2 3 4

Picture 8. Typisation of *B. burgdorferi* s.l.genospecies of isolates by PCR technique: species specific PCR for *B. burgdorferi* s.l. isolates; M: DNA size marker specific fragment 50bp; 1:Pool „244"isolate amplified with specific primers for *B. burgdorferi sensu stricto*; 2-4: Pools „Granicar 1 and 2"andi „Novi Sad" isolates amplified with specific primers for *B. afzelii*

6.1 Statistics – Kappa test

Data gathered during the research was analysed by Kappa statistic test (Valčić 1998). This test is useful for the analysis of methods which as a result have „posotove-negative" values, instead of numeric values. Statistical analysis with Kappa method is used for comparing of compatibility of findings among two tests or methods. Kappa value 1 is for a complete and ideal comatibility and 0 is for a accidental compatibility of tests. All the other values can be in between. Compatibility of methods Western blot and ELISA for serological findings in three groups of dogs is 0,915, meaning that the compatibility of these two methods is ideal. Compatibility of fast test and ELISA (or Western blot, because the values were the same for those two tests) for serological findings in second group of dogs after natural infection, is also high, its 1, maening that the compatibility of methods is ideal or complete. CF method does not have complete compability compared to ELISA or Western blott. This means that ELISA or Western blott can be eaqualy used in diagnostics of Lyme disease.

6.2 Resume of Lyme disease in ticks and dogs in Serbia

In Serbia, research on ticks as vectors of infectious agents started over 60 years ago. Lyme disease was discovered in 1987, and more intensive research on ticks, their ecology, seasonality... Over the years there have been some changes becauseof the changes and irregularities in climate and metrology factors. Reaserch done in the last several years in Serbia have prooved infection in I. ricinus ticsk with *B. burgdorferi* between 20 - 30% (Milutinović et all, 2004; Jurišić, 2008; Cekanac et all, 2009), and in some parts even over 40% (Milutinović et all, 2008). During this three year period of research in chosen localities an average infection of ticks with *B. burgdorferi* s.l. is 22,12%. The highest percentage of infected ticks was found to be in urban region with surrounding (29,2%) and in one locality (in Banat region), there were no infected ticks found at all.

The average value of ERI found in this research was 0,033. The highest risk from Lyme disease was found to be in urbane region with surroundings (0,053), where also was highest rate of ticks infected with *B. burgdorferi* s.l. In literature it is mentioned that the value of ERI is in correlation with the number of human cases with Lyme disease. Calculated value of ERI in a region can be useful information in estimation of the risk from spreading of Lyme disease in a certain region and also for the prediction of appearance of Lyme disease in humans (Mather et all, 1996).

From the ticks collected in the region, four autochthonous strains of *B. burgdorferi* s.l. were isolated and three of those strains belonged to genospecies *B. afzelii,* and one belonged to genospecies *B. burgdorferi sensu stricto*. Several authors worked on isolation of Borrelia from ticks and their identification and typisation to the genospecies level with method based on PCR technology (Cerar et al 2009, Lindblom et all 2009, Wilhelmsson et all 2009). Results on the outspread of *B. burgdorferi* genospecies in vectors of Lyme disease show a dominant presence of *B. afzelii,* compared to a less frequent occurrence of *B. burgdorferi sensu stricto* in ticks. Additionally, the findings after analysis done with Western blot highlight the same result: from the total of 127 dogs with a seropositive serology finding for *B. burgdorferi,* in 107 dogs, the presence of specific antibodies to protein antigens characteristic for *B. afzelii* were found. In previous research done in the region of Serbia (different localities), the domination of *B. afzelii* was also found, compared to *B. burgdorferi sensu stricto* and *B. garinii* (Cekanac et all, 2009).

Clinical symptoms were found in a certain number of dogs. Since in most of the dogs specific antibodies against antigens of genospecies B. *afzelii* were confirmed, it can be stated that in Serbia region where the research was done, cases of Lyme disease in dogs is mostly caused by *B. afzelii* with general clinical symptoms of difficult moving, lameness, lethargy, irregular elevation of body temperature up to 40°C, loss of appetite and weakness. Two groups of dogs were analyzed which did not have clinical symptoms that could be related to Lyme disease and a prevalence was found for *B. burgdorferi* s.l. In group of dogs used as working, hunting and military dogs the prevalence was in the range from 21 - 37%, depending on the laboratory method used and in the group of dogs which were kept as pets the prevalence for *B. burgdorferi* was in the range from 26 - 33%. The prevalence found in one group of dogs was not much different than in the other, even though one group is constantly exposed to the tick influence, so the risk from occurrence of the disease is pretty much the same no matter if dogs are being used for hunting or as pets, as long as they are protected by antiectoparasitic products.

A significant difference in the percentage of positive findings during the research was gained, related to the method used for diagnostic, in dogs with Lyme disease. Author Jovičić in her research concludes that ELISA test should be used at the beginning of diagnostic process in humans suspicious for Lyme borreliosis and Western blott is to be used as conformation method (Jovičić, 2001). The findings from this research pretty much backup this statement. In this research, in dogs with clinical symptoms of Lyme disease , the greatest number of positive serology findings was gained by CF method (93,75% of positive samples). But far more balanced and unified results were found by ELISA (87,5% positive samples), Western blot (87,5% positive samples) and fast test (81,25% positive samples). CF method in diagnostic of Lyme disease can only be used as „screening" method for research purposes and in everyday routine this method is nor useful. Fast tests can be used for first glance diagnostic, for fast and orientational result. If there is a dog with clinical symptoms that could indicate to Lyme disease, fast tests should always be used as first method. Every positive finding should be confirmed by another method like ELISA or Western blot. If fast test gives a negative result and there is still a suspicion of Lyme disease, analysis should be repeated with a more sensitive method (ELISA or Western blot) in a certain time interval, for a more complete and confident diagnosis. Several authors recognize ELISA as the most convenient method for monitoring and clinical check up of Lyme disease in dog population, because it is a highly sensitive test with objectivity in resulting (Magnarelli et all, 1988, Goosens et all, 2000). Western blott is often described by the authors as conformation method and proteins of molecular weight in the range from 66-73 kDa (in this research VIsE from 66kDa was used) are considered to be dominant immunogenes present in every pathogen genospecies of *B. burgdorferi sensu lato* (Luft et all, 1991). In this research by Western blott method in the majority of positive samples for Lyme disease, antibodies for protein antigens of genospecies *B. afzelii* were detected (84%).

In dogs that did not have clinical symptoms indicating Lyme disease an "accidental" positive finding should be interpreted very carefully, having in mind all the relevant data for making a definite diagnosis. There are fast tests that can diagnose few diseases at once like fast test for erlichiosis, dirofilariosis and borreliosis. Usage of these tests can mislead in diagnosis if initially there is a suspicious for another disease and the test gives a positive result for Lyme disease. Serology testing for Lyme disease does not have any value in predicting the condition in limbs or joints (Levy and Magnarelli, 1992.). For exact diagnosis it always has to be asked if dog has spent some time in a region which is endemic for Lyme borreliosis. After infection, 4-6 weeks is needed for immunoresponse and before this period is over, a negative serology result can be found even if a dog is infected. Diagnosis in Lyme disease has to be done based on epizootiological anamnesis, clinical check up and laboratory analysis.

7. Acknowledgments

This work is supported by a grant from the Ministry of Research and Technological Development, Republic of Serbia, Project number TR 31071

8. References

[1] Burgdorfer W, Hayes SF, Corwin D: „Pathophysiology of the Lyme disease spirchete, Borrelia burgdorferi, in ixodid ticks", Review of infectious diseases, Sept-Oct, suppl 6, 1442-1450, 1989.

[2] Burgdorfer W: „Lyme borreliosis: ten years after discovery of the etiologic agent, Borrelia burgdorferi", Infection, Jul-Aug, 19 (4), 257-262, 1991.

[3] Cekanac R, Pavlović N, Gledović Z, Grgurević A, Stajković N, Lepsanovic Z, Ristanović E: „Prevalence of *Borrelia burgdorferi* in *Ixodes ricinus* ticks in Belgrade area", Vector Borne Zoonotic Disease, Dec 18, (Epub ahead of print) 2009.

[4] Cerar T, Ferdin J, Strle F, Zore A, Ružić-Sabljić E: „Real time PCR based on HBB gene for identification of Borrelia burgdorfei sensu lato", Proceedings of FEMS, 3rd Congress of European microbiologists, Sweden, 2009.

[5] Cisak E, Wojcik-Fatla A, Stojek N.M, Chmielewska-Badora J, Zwolonski J, Buczek A, Dutkiewicz J: „Prevalence of Borrelia burgdorferi genospecies in *Ixodes ricinus* ticks from Lublin region (eastern Poland)", Ann Agric Environ Med, 13, 301-306, 2006.

[6] Dmitrović R, Popović N: „Lajmska bolest", Veterinarski glasnik 1-2, Vol 47, 59-63, 1993.

[7] Duncan AW, Correa MT, Levine JF, Breitschwerdt EB: „The dog as sentinel for human infection: prevalence of Borrelia burgdorferi C6 antibodies in dogs from southeastern and mid Atlantic States", Vector borne Zoonotic Diseases, 5(2), 101-109, 2005.

[8] Epidemiological bullitein: „Lyme borreliosis, 30 years after", No 72, year VIII, may, 2005.

[9] Golubić D, Rijpkema S, Tkalec-Makovec N, Ružić E: „Epidemiologic, ecologic and clinical characteristics of Lyme disease in northwest Croatia", Acta Medica Croatica, 52 (1), 7-13, 1998.

[10] Goosens HA, van der Bogaard AE, Nohlmans MK: „Reduced specificity of comined IgM and IgG enzyme immunoassay testing for lyme borreliosis", European Journal of Clinical Microbiology and Infectious diseases, 19, 5, 400-402, 2000.

[11] Hulinska D, Votypka J, Kriz B, Holinkova N, Novakova J, Hulinsky V: „Phenotypic and genotypic analysis of Borrelia spp. Isolated from Ixodes ricinus ticks by using electrofortic chips and real-time polimerasa polymerase chain reaction", Folia Mikrobiol, 52 (4), 315-24, 2007.

[12] Jacobson RH, Chang ZF, Shin SJ: Lyme disease: „Laboratory diagnostics of infected and vaccinated symptomatic dogs", Proceedings of Seminar of Veterinary Medicine Surgery (Small Animal), Aug, 11 (3), 172-182, 1996.

[13] Jovičić V: „Savremena dijagnostika lajmske borelioze", monografija, Biblioteka Dissertatio, Zadužbina Andrejević, Beograd, 2001.

[14] Jurišić A., Magistarska teza: „Fauna krpelja i njihov značaj kao vektora uzročnika lajmske bolesti u urbanoj sredini", Univerzitet u Novom Sadu, Poljoprivredni fakultet, Novi Sad, 2005.

[15] Jurišić A: „Krpelji-prenosioci uzročnika bolesti kod ljudi i životinja", monografija, Biblioteka Akademia, Zadužbina Andrejević, Beograd, 2008.

[16] Lako B, Dmitrović R, Drndarević D, Nanušević N, Lazarević N, Obradović M, Đorđević D: „Our first experiances with serological diagnosis of Lyme disease", IX jugoslovensko-italijanski sastanak o zaraznim bolestima, Beograd, Abstracts, 45, 1998.

[17] Levy SA, Lissman BA, Ficke CM: „Performance of a Borrelia burgdorferi bacterin in borreliosis-endemic areas", Journal of American Veterinary Medicine Assosiation, Jun 1, 202(11), 1834-1838, 1993.

[18] Levy SA, Magnarelli LA: „Relationship between development of antibodies to Borrelia burgdorferi in dogs and the susequent development of limb/joint borreliosis",

Journal of American Veterinary Medicine Assosiation, February 1, 200(3), 344-347, 1992.

[19] Lindblom P, Wilhelmsson P, Fryland L, Jansson C, Carlsson S.A, ny,an D, Ekerfelt C, Ernerudh J, Forsberg P, Lindgren P.E: „Epidemiological study of tick-borne pathogens in Sweden and Aland - prevelancein ticks detached from humans connected to risk of developing symptomatic and asymptomatic infection", Proceedings of FEMS, 3rd Congress of European microbiologists, Sweden, 2009.

[20] Lindgren E, Jaenson TGT: „Lyme borreliosis in Europe: influence of climate and climate change, epidemiology, ecology and adaptation measures", Projekat Stokholm Univerziteta i World Health Organisation, Regional Office for Europe, pod pokroviteljstvom European Commission, 2004.

[21] Lopes de Carvalho I, Nuncio MS: „Laboratory diagnosis of Lyme borreliosis at the Portuguese National Institute of health (1990-2004), Eurosurveillance, Vol 11, Iss 10, 2006.

[22] Luft BJ, Gorević PD, Jiang W, Munoz P, Dattwyler RJ: „Immunologic and stuctural characterization of the dominant 66-to 73-kDa antigens of Borrelia burgdorferi", Journal of Immunology, 146(8), 2776-2782, 1991.

[23] Magnarelli L.A, Anderson J.F, Hyland K.E, Fish D, Mcaninch J.B: „Serologic analyses of Peromyscus leucopus, a rodent reservoair for Borrelia burgdorferi in Northeastern United States", Journal of clinical microbiology, Vol 26, No 6, 1138-1141, 1988.

[24] Mather TN, Nicholson MC, Donnelly EF, Matyas BT: „Entomologic index for human risk of Lyme disease, American Journal of Epidemiology, 144 (11), 1066-1069, 1996.

[25] Merino FJ, Nebreda T, Serrano JL, Fernandez-Soto P, Encinas A, Perez-Sanchez R: „ Tick species and tick-borne infections identified in population from a rural area of Spain", Epidemiology and Infectology, 133(5), 943-949, 2005.

[26] Merino FJ, Serrano JL, Saz JV, Nebreda T, Gegundez M, Beltran M: „Epidemiological characteristics of dogs with Lyme borreliosis in the province of Soria (Spain)", European Journal of Epidemiology, 16(2), 97-100, 2000.

[27] Milutinović M, Masuzawa T, Tomanović S, Radulović Ž, Fukui T, Okamoto Y: *„Borrelia burgdorferi* sensu lato, *Anaplasma phagocytophilum, Francisella tularensis* and their co-infections in host seeking *Ixodes ricinus* ticks collected in Serbia", Exp Applied Acarology, 45, 171-183, 2008.

[28] Milutinović M, Radulović Ž, Jovičić V, Oreščanin Z: „Population dynamics and Borrelia burgdorferi infection rate of Ixodes ricinus ticks in the Belgrade area", Acta Veterinaria, Vol 54, No 2-3, 219-225, 2004.

[29] Moran Cadenas F, Rais O, Humair PF, Douet V, Moret J, Gern L: „Identification of host bloodmeal source and Borrelia burgdorferi sensu lato in field-collected Ixodes ricinus ticks in Chaumont (Switzerland)", Journal of Medical Entomology, 44(6), 1109-1117, 2007.

[30] Pejchalova K, Žakovska A, Mejzlikova M, Halouzka J, Dendis M: „Isolation, cultivaton and identification of Borrelia burgdorferi genospecies from Ixodes ricinus ticks from the city of Brno", Czech republic; Ann Agric Environ Med, 14, 75-79, 2007.

[31] Savić-Jevđenić S, Grgić, Ž, Vidić B, Petrovi- A: „Lyme disease - the great imitator", Biotechnology in animal husbandry, Vol 23, 5-6, 215-221, 2007.

[32] Savić-Jevđenić S, Vidić B, Grgić Ž, Jurišić A, Lako B: „Lyme borreliosis in hunting dogs", Book of Proceedings, VI international Conference on ticks and tick-borne pathogens, TTP-6, Buenos Aires, Argentina, pg 317, 2008.

[33] Schulze TL, Bosler EM, Shisler JK, Ware IC, Lakat MF, Parkin WE: „Prevalence of canine Lyme disease from an endemic area as determined by serosurvey", Zentralbl Bakteriol Mikrobiol Hyg, 263 (3), 427-424, 1987.

[34] Skotarczak B: „Lyme borreliosis in dogs", knjiga Peter van Nitch: „Research on Lyme disease", Nova Science Publishers, Inc, 69-81, 2007.

[35] Valčić M.A: „Opšta epizootiologija", Univerzitet u Beogradu, Fakultet veterinarske medicine, Beograd, 1998.

[36] Wall R, Shearer D: „Veterinary Entomology", Chapman and Hall, London, Ticks 97-140, 1992.

[37] Wilhelmsson P, Fryland L, Borjesson S, Nordgren J, Ekerfelt C, Ernerudh J, Forsberg P, Lindgren P.E: „Detection, quantification, and genotyping of Borrelia-spirochetes from ticks that have bitten humans", Proceedings of FEMS, 3rd Congress of European microbiologists, Sweden, 2009.

[38] Wright JC, Chambers M, Mullen GR, Swango LJ, D'Andrea GH, Boyce AJ: "Seroprevalance of Borrelia burgdorferi in dogs in Alabama, USA", Preventive Veterinary Medicine, 31(1-2), 127-131, 1997.

[39] Zuckert WR: „Laboratory Maintance of Borrelia burgdorferi", Current Protocols in Mycrobiology, Copyright 2007 by John Wiley & Sons, Inc, 12C1.1. - 12C1.10, 2007.

6

Adaptation to Glucosamine Starvation in *Borrelia burgdorferi* is Mediated by *recA*

Ryan G. Rhodes[1], Janet A. Atoyan[2] and David R. Nelson[2]
[1]*St. Bonaventure University, St. Bonaventure, NY*
[2]*University of Rhode Island, Kingston, RI*
USA

1. Introduction

Lyme borreliosis is a vector-borne disease confined primarily to the Northern hemisphere and caused by spirochetes belonging to the *Borrelia burgdorferi* sensu lato (s.l.) genospecies (Kurtenbach et al. 2006). The spirochetes are maintained exclusively within an enzootic cycle, alternating between a tick vector and vertebrate host. *B. burgdorferi* s.l. includes three pathogenic species and at least eight related species that are non-pathogenic or rarely cause infection in humans. The three pathogenic species include *B. burgdorferi* sensu stricto (s.s.), the only species found in North America, and *B. garinii* and *B. afzelii* the causative agents of borreliosis in Europe and Asia (Steere et al. 2004). These three species cause similar acute and chronic illness in humans, although regional differences do exist (Steere 2001).

B. burgdorferi is a limited genome organism and must scavenge most essential nutrients from its tick vector or vertebrate host (Das 2000; Saier MH 2000). The organism requires a complex medium for propagation in the laboratory, and specific addition of free N-acetyl-glucosamine (GlcNAc), a component of the bacterial cell wall, is necessary for cells to reach optimal cell densities in a single exponential phase (Barbour 1984; Tilly et al. 2001; Rhodes et al. 2009; Rhodes et al. 2010). In the absence of free GlcNAc *B. burgdorferi* can degrade chitin (a polymer of GlcNAc) to chitobiose and import this dimer through a dedicated chitobiose phosphotransferase system to satisfy its requirement for exogenous GlcNAc (Rhodes et al. 2010). However, in the absence of both free GlcNAc and chitin this spirochete exhibits a unique biphasic growth pattern in which the second exponential phase is dependent on the expression of the chitobiose transporter (Tilly et al. 2001; Rhodes et al. 2009; Rhodes et al. 2010). In the first exponential phase cells grow to approximately 2.0×10^6 cells ml^{-1} within three days by exhausting the small amount of free GlcNAc and/or GlcNAc oligomers from complex medium components such as rabbit serum and yeastolate. After utilizing these sources of GlcNAc cells exhibit a death phase in which cell density decreases below 1.0×10^5 cells ml^{-1} between days three and five. Finally, a second exponential phase is initiated between days five and seven in which cells grow to near optimal cell density ($\sim 5.0 \times 10^7$ cells ml^{-1}).

This peculiar growth pattern in the absence of free GlcNAc or chitin suggests there is a sequestered (or bound) source of GlcNAc within the medium that cells can access in the second exponential phase, but are unable to utilize in the first exponential phase. While this source remains unknown, as well as the mechanism(s) used to obtain it, our data demonstrating the utilization of chitin by *B. burgdorferi* in the absence of free GlcNAc suggests that polymerized GlcNAc is not the source (Rhodes et al. 2010). In addition, it is unclear whether the adaptation to GlcNAc starvation (i.e. second exponential phase growth) is physiologic or genetic in nature. A previous report by Tilly et al. (Tilly et al. 2001) suggested that second exponential phase growth was a physiologic response, as cells from the second exponential phase exhibited biphasic growth after being transferred to fresh medium lacking GlcNAc. However, in that experiment starvation-adapted cells grew almost 10-fold higher in the first exponential phase as compared to cells that were not previously exposed to the starvation condition, leaving open the possibility that second exponential phase growth is due to the outgrowth of a mutant population.

Stress-induced mutagenesis occurring in bacteria under growth-limiting conditions is a phenomenon that has been intensively studied in recent years. Nearly two decades ago Cairns and Foster described adaptive reversion using an *Escherichia coli* Lac assay (Cairns & Foster 1991). In this system cells carrying a *lacI-lacZ* fusion gene with a +1 frameshift mutation in *lacI* were unable to utilize lactose, but when cultured with a non-lactose carbon source and then spread onto lactose plates, Lac+ revertants were obtained. Characterization of these stress-induced mutants revealed they were of two types: i) point mutants carrying a compensatory frameshift mutation in *lac* (Foster & Trimarchi 1994; Rosenberg et al. 1994) or ii) *lac*-amplified cells in which the leaky *lac* frameshift allele was amplified 20-50 times (Hastings et al. 2000; Powell & Wartell 2001; Kugelberg et al. 2006; Slack et al. 2006). Substantial work has been conducted to elucidate the underlying molecular mechanisms responsible for these two distinct types of stress-induced mutants. Formation of the Lac+ point mutants can occur via several stress-response and DNA repair and metabolism pathways, including i) homologous recombination via double-strand-break-repair (DSBR) proteins (Cairns & Foster 1991; Harris et al. 1994), ii) error-prone DNA replication (McKenzie et al. 2001), iii) the SOS response (McKenzie et al. 2000), iv) the RpoS starvation-stress response (Lombardo et al. 2004), and v) methyl-directed mismatch repair (MMR) (Harris et al. 1999). In contrast, *lac*-amplification does not require error-prone DNA replication or the SOS response (McKenzie et al. 2001), but does require the general stress-response regulator RpoS and homologous recombination via DSBR proteins such as RecA, RecBCD and RuvABC (Slack et al. 2006). While *B. burgdorferi* has a limited genome and lacks error-prone DNA polymerases and the SOS pathway, it is possible that stress-induced mutagenesis occurs in this organism and could be mediated by mismatch repair, RpoS and/or homologous recombination.

Several studies have been conducted in *B. burgdorferi* to evaluate the function of RecA both *in vitro* and *in vivo* (Liveris et al. 2004; Putteet-Driver et al. 2004; Liveris et al. 2008). Early attempts to generate a *recA* null mutant were unsuccessful; therefore transgenic expression of *B. burgdorferi* RecA in *E. coli* was used to determine its functional properties (Liveris et al. 2004; Putteet-Driver et al. 2004). In *E. coli* RecA has three major activities: i) it participates in homologous recombination by catalyzing DNA strand exchange, ii) it promotes the autocatalytic cleavage of LexA, a repressor of the SOS response, and iii) it directly facilitates bypass of DNA lesions by DNA polymerase V during the SOS response (Cox 2007). Complementation of an *E. coli recA* null mutant with *B. burgdorferi recA* restored the ability of the mutant to promote homologous recombination and activated the *E. coli* SOS pathway in response to DNA-damaging agents (Liveris et al. 2004; Putteet-Driver et al. 2004). In a more recent study, Liveris *et al* (Liveris et al. 2008) successfully generated a *recA* mutant in a low passage infectious *B. burgdorferi* strain and showed that RecA mediates homologous recombination in this organism. However, this report demonstrated RecA is only minimally involved in DNA repair in response to DNA damaging agents, and does not mediate antigenic variation at the *vlsE* locus after mammalian infection.

As described above, a previous attempt to characterize *B. burgdorferi* second exponential phase growth in the absence of free GlcNAc has left unanswered questions as to whether this is a physiologic or genetic adaptation to the starvation condition. In this study we follow the growth of wild-type and *recA* mutant cells in the absence of free GlcNAc and suggest that growth in the second exponential phase is the result of a genetic adaptation that is, at least in part, mediated by RecA. Additionally, we characterize the *recA* transcriptional unit and provide evidence suggesting this gene is transcribed from two separate promoters.

2. Results

2.1 Adaptation to GlcNAc starvation

Wild-type cells cultured in the absence of free GlcNAc exhibit biphasic growth (Fig. 1A), with growth in the second exponential phase dependent on the expression of the chitobiose transporter *chbC* (Tilly et al. 2001; Rhodes et al. 2010). To determine if cells in the second exponential phase were adapted to grow in the absence of free GlcNAc we followed cell growth in BSK-II lacking GlcNAc. Cells were diluted to 1.0×10^5 cells ml^{-1} in the same medium at various time points along the biphasic growth curve, and growth of the new cultures was followed to determine if biphasic growth occurred (Fig. 1B and C). Diluting cells during the first exponential phase on day 2 (46 h) or at the peak of the first exponential phase on day 3 (72 h) into BSK-II lacking GlcNAc resulted in biphasic growth (Fig. 1B). In contrast, cells diluted from the second exponential phase on days 8-11 (191, 216, 237 and 263 h) into BSK-II lacking GlcNAc resulted in growth to high cell densities in a single exponential phase, with cell densities reaching $\geq 2.5 \times 10^7$ cells ml^{-1} (Fig. 1C). This cell density is equivalent to that reached by cells in the second exponential phase when cultured in BSK-II lacking free GlcNAc, though about one-tenth the cell densities reached by cells cultured in complete BSK-II. In some experiments cells diluted from the second exponential phase were followed for extended periods of time after reaching their peak cell density ($\sim 2.5 \times 10^7$ cells ml^{-1}) in a single exponential phase, and while there was a decline in cell density a second exponential phase was not observed as previously described (Tilly et al. 2001).

2.2 Adaptation to GlcNAc is the result of a mutational event

Two possible explanations for second exponential phase growth in a GlcNAc depleted medium are that: 1) second exponential phase growth occurs as a result of a physiological adaptation to GlcNAc starvation as cells induce genes to utilize sequestered GlcNAc; or that 2) second exponential phase growth occurs as the result of a mutational event that allows for the outgrowth of a mutant population able to obtain sequestered GlcNAc from a source they were previously unable to utilize. If second exponential phase growth was the result of a mutational event, it would be expected that cells removed from the second exponential phase would retain the ability to grow in a single exponential phase in BSK-II lacking

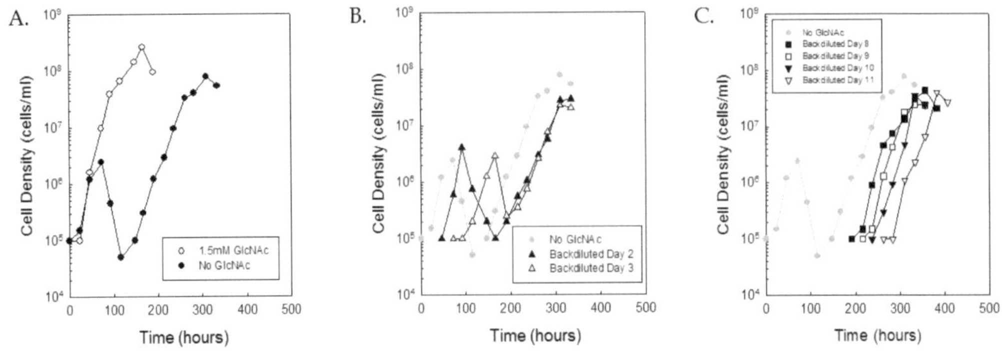

Fig. 1. Adaptation of B31-A to GlcNAc starvation. (A) Growth of B31-A in BSK-II with and without 1.5mM GlcNAc. Late-log phase cells were diluted to 1.0×10^5 cells ml^{-1} in complete BSK-II (open circle) or BSK-II lacking GlcNAc (closed circle), and cells were enumerated daily by darkfield microscopy. (B) Growth of B31-A in BSK-II without GlcNAc after dilution from the first exponential phase of a culture starved for GlcNAc. Cells starved for GlcNAc (closed gray circle) were diluted to 1.0×10^5 cells ml^{-1} at day 2 (closed triangle) and day 3 (open triangle) into BSK-II without GlcNAc, and growth was followed daily by darkfield microscopy. (C) Growth of B31-A in BSK-II without GlcNAc after dilution from the second exponential phase of a culture starved for GlcNAc. Cells starved for GlcNAc (closed gray circle) were diluted to 1.0×10^5 cells ml^{-1} at day 8 (closed square), day 9 (open square), day 10 (inverted closed triangle) and day 11 (inverted open triangle) into BSK-II without GlcNAc, and growth was followed daily by darkfield microscopy. These growth curves are representative of four independent growth experiments.

GlcNAc after serial passage in complete BSK-II. On the other hand, if a physiologic mechanism was responsible, then it would be expected that cells removed from the second exponential phase and subjected to serial passage in a complete medium would still exhibit biphasic growth when transferred back to a medium lacking GlcNAc. To test this, cells were diluted from the second exponential phase into complete BSK-II, serially passaged up to twelve times in this complete medium, and then re-evaluated for biphasic growth after being transferred back to BSK-II lacking GlcNAc (Fig. 2). Despite being cultured in the presence of free GlcNAc for up to twelve passages, cells exhibited only one exponential phase upon re-introduction to BSK-II lacking GlcNAc. Interestingly, cells diluted into BSK-II without GlcNAc after 7 and 12 serial passages in complete BSK-II grew to a higher cell density (~5-fold) than cells cultured in complete BSK-II for 1 or 2 passages.

To further demonstrate that adaptation to GlcNAc starvation is the result of a genetic event, cells were plated on BSK-II agar and the growth of wild-type or starvation-adapted clones was followed. Specifically, wild-type cells cultured in complete BSK-II and starvation-adapted cells serially passaged seven times in complete BSK-II (P. 7 No GlcNAc from Fig. 2; closed squares) were plated on BSK-II agar containing free GlcNAc to obtain isolated colonies. Ten clones from each were transferred to BSK-II broth lacking GlcNAc and growth was followed daily. All ten clones from wild-type cells not previously adapted to GlcNAc starvation exhibited biphasic growth when cultured in the absence of free GlcNAc (Fig. 3A). In contrast, eight of the ten clones obtained from cells previously adapted to GlcNAc starvation and serially passaged seven times in complete BSK-II grew to optimal cell densities in a single exponential phase when cultured in BSK-II lacking free GlcNAc (Fig. 3B).

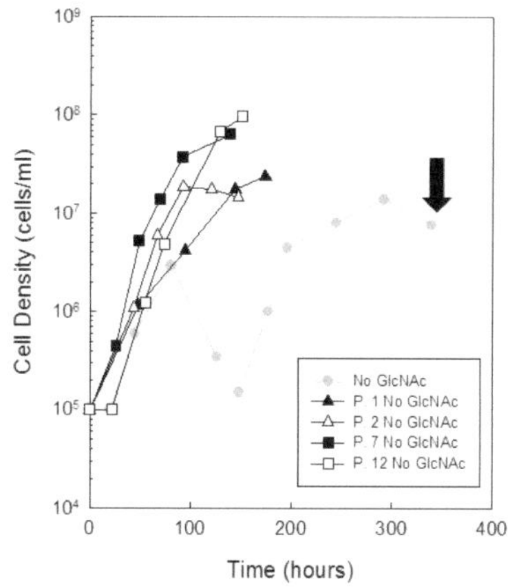

Fig. 2. Growth of starvation-adapted cells in BSK-II without GlcNAc after repeated subculture in complete BSK-II. B31-A cells grown in BSK-II without added GlcNAc (closed gray circle) were transferred (arrow indicates point at which adapted cells were sub-cultured) to complete BSK-II. After one passage in complete BSK-II cells were diluted to 1.0 × 10^5 cells ml^{-1} in BSK-II without GlcNAc (P. 1; closed triangle) and growth was followed daily by darkfield microscopy. Growth was also followed in BSK-II without GlcNAc after two (P. 2; open triangle), seven (P. 7; closed square) and twelve (P. 12; open square) serial passages in complete BSK-II. This is a representative experiment that was repeated twice.

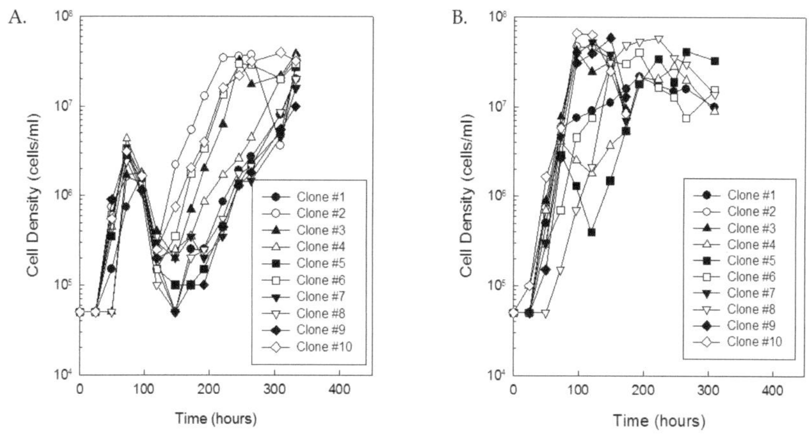

Fig. 3. Growth of GlcNAc starvation adapted and non-adapted clones in BSK-II without GlcNAc. (A) B31-A cells cultured in complete BSK-II (non-adapted) were plated on BSK-II agar (containing GlcNAc) and 10 clones were transferred to BSK-II broth without GlcNAc. Growth was followed daily by darkfield microscopy. (B) B31-A cells adapted to GlcNAc starvation and serially passaged in complete BSK-II were plated on solid medium and 10 clones were transferred to liquid BSK-II without GlcNAc. Growth was followed daily by darkfield microscopy.

It is possible that the two clones (clones #4 and #5 from Fig. 3B) from GlcNAc starvation-adapted cells exhibited biphasic growth as the result of a second-site mutation or it may be that a sub-population of non-adapted cells was able to persist in the absence of GlcNAc as the result of the mutant population releasing sequestered GlcNAc from an as yet unknown medium component. In an attempt to clarify this point, cells from starvation-adapted clone #10 (Fig. 3B; designated RR45) were passaged twice in complete BSK-II, and then plated on BSK-II agar with GlcNAc. Ten clones were transferred to BSK-II broth without GlcNAc and growth was followed daily by darkfield microscopy. In addition, wild-type cells cultured in complete BSK-II were plated on BSK-II agar with GlcNAc, and the growth of ten clones was followed in liquid BSK-II without GlcNAc (Fig. 4A). As previously demonstrated, the ten wild-type clones exhibited biphasic growth (Fig. 4A). In contrast, all ten RR45 clones grew to optimal cell densities in a single exponential phase (Fig. 4B).

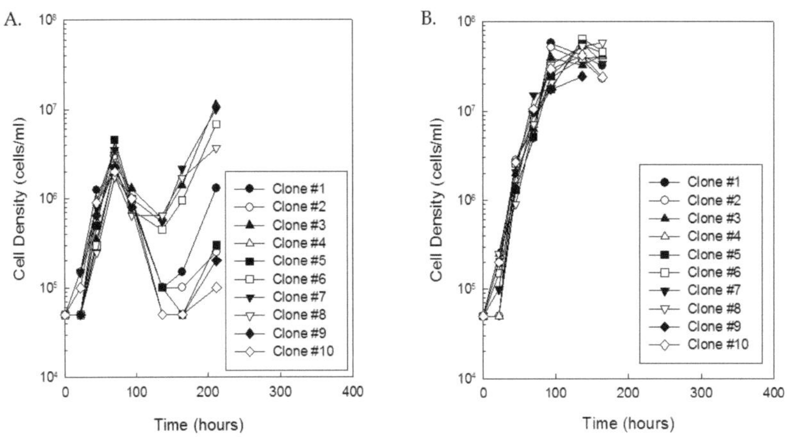

Fig. 4. Growth of GlcNAc starvation adapted RR45 and non-adapted wild-type clones in BSK-II without GlcNAc. (A) B31-A cells cultured in complete BSK-II (non-adapted) were plated on complete BSK-II agar and 10 clones were transferred to liquid BSK-II without GlcNAc. Growth was followed daily by darkfield microscopy. (B) RR45 cells (clone #10 from Fig. 3B) were plated on complete BSK-II agar and 10 clones were transferred to liquid BSK-II without GlcNAc. Growth was followed daily by darkfield microscopy.

2.3 Construction and characterization of a *B. burgdorferi recA* mutant and two complemented mutants

As double-strand-break-repair (DSBR) proteins, such as RecA, have been shown to be involved in stress-induced mutation in *E. coli* (He et al. 2006), we hypothesized that *recA* may play a role in the ability of *B. burgdorferi* to adapt to GlcNAc starvation. Therefore, we generated a *recA* deletion mutant in the B31-A background by allelic exchange, and designated this strain JA10 (see Methods). To confirm that RecA function was inactivated, we examined survival after exposure to DNA-damaging agents, as well as the ability to promote homologous recombination. Recently, Liveris et al. (Liveris et al. 2008) demonstrated that a low-passage infectious *B. burgdorferi recA* mutant was only moderately sensitive to DNA-damaging agents (UV irradiation and mitomycin C), but showed that RecA was essential for allelic exchange in this organism. We confirmed those results here using a high-passage non-infectious *recA* mutant (JA10) which showed no significant difference in sensitivity to DNA-damaging agents when compared to wild-type cells (data not shown), but was unable to promote homologous recombination (Table 1). Recombination frequency was determined by transforming each strain with pBB0450.1

Strain	Transformation Frequency[a]		Recombination Frequency[b]	
	n[c]	Average (±SD)	*n*[d]	Average (±SD)
B31-A	4	6.7×10^{-5} ($\pm 7.2 \times 10^{-5}$)	5	3.3×10^{-6} ($\pm 1.8 \times 10^{-6}$)
JA10	3	5.4×10^{-5} ($\pm 7.5 \times 10^{-5}$)	5	0 (± 0)
JA15	2	5.6×10^{-5} (ND[e])	4	0 (± 0)
JR1	7	3.4×10^{-7} ($\pm 2.6 \times 10^{-7}$)	7	6.5×10^{-6} ($\pm 1.2 \times 10^{-5}$)

[a] Transformation frequency is the number of transformants obtained after electroporation of cells with ErmC/pCE320 divided by the number of CFU obtained without antibiotic selection
[b] Recombination frequency is the number of recombinants obtained after electroporation of cells with pBB0450.1 (*rpoN::ermC*) divided by the number of CFU obtained without antibiotic selection
[c] Number of transformation experiments performed with ErmC/pCE320 to determine transformation frequency.
[d] Number of transformation experiments performed with pBB0450.1 to determine recombination frequency.
[e] ND, Not determined

Table 1. Transformation and recombination frequencies of the wild type (B31-A), *recA* mutant (JA10) and *recA* complemented mutants (JA15 and JR1).

(*ermC::rpoN*), a suicide vector carrying a mutant *rpoN* allele that confers erythromycin resistance. The wild-type strain exhibited a recombination frequency of 3.3×10^{-6} (Table 1), while no recombinants were observed for the *recA* mutant. It is possible, though unlikely, that the lack of recombination observed in the *recA* mutant was due to the inability of the plasmid to gain entry into the cell during electroporation. Therefore, we determined the transformation frequency of all strains by modifying the pCE320 *B. burgdorferi* shuttle vector to confer erythromycin resistance, and transformed cells with this new plasmid designated ErmC/pCE320. Transformation frequency was similar for both the wild-type and *recA* mutant strains (6.7×10^{-5} and 5.4×10^{-5}, respectively; Table 1), suggesting that the lack of recombinants observed after transformation with pBB0450.1 was due to the absence of a functional *recA* gene.

To provide further evidence that the *recA* gene in JA10 was inactivated, the mutant was complemented with plasmid pBB0131comp.2 which consists of the wild-type *recA* gene with 512 bp of upstream DNA, presumably encompassing its natural promoter, cloned into the *B. burgdorferi* shuttle vector pBSV2 (see Methods). This strain was designated JA15 and transformation and recombination frequencies were determined as described above. The JA15 complemented mutant exhibited a transformation frequency similar to that observed for the wild-type and *recA* mutant strains (5.6×10^{-5}; Table 1). However, this strain unexpectedly exhibited no homologous recombination, suggesting the 512 bp of DNA upstream of the *recA* translational start site may not be sufficient for expression of *recA* at wild-type levels. Therefore, we generated a second *recA* complemented mutant using plasmid pRecA.3 consisting of the wild-type *recA* gene fused to the constitutive *B. burgdorferi flaB* promoter and cloned into the shuttle vector pCE320. This strain was designated JR1 and transformation and recombination frequencies were determined. While this strain exhibited a marked reduction in transformation frequency compared to the wild-type strain, RecA function was restored as JR1 demonstrated a 2-fold greater recombination frequency as compared to B31-A (Table 1). The reduction in transformation frequency observed in JR1 is likely due to the incompatibility of pRecA.3 and ErmC/pCE320 as they are both derivatives of the pCE320 shuttle vector.

2.4 Expression of *recA* determined by quantitative RT-PCR (qRT-PCR)

One possible explanation for the lack of recombination observed in the JA15 strain is that *recA* transcription was reduced, leading to decreased levels of functional RecA protein. To test this, we evaluated *recA* expression in B31-A, JA10, JA15 and JR1 using qRT-PCR (Table 2). RNA was extracted from late-log phase cells (~2.0×10^7 cells ml^{-1}) and the amount of *recA* transcript present in 10 ng of total RNA was determined. As expected, *recA* transcript levels in the JA15 complemented mutant were 61.5-fold lower than those measured in wild-type cells, possibly accounting for the lack of recombination observed in this strain. In contrast, *recA* transcript levels in the JR1 complemented mutant, in which *recA* expression was driven by a constitutive promoter, were 15.7-fold higher than the wild type. No *recA* transcription was detected in JA10 cells. These results may explain the 2-fold increase observed in recombination frequency in JR1 compared to the wild type. It is important to note that despite the differences in *recA* levels in these different strains, the growth rate between strains did not vary and the growth curves in complete BSK-II were indistinguishable (data not shown).

Strain	*recA* Copy Number Average[a] (±SD[b])	Fold Difference[c]
B31-A	8.49×10^5 ($\pm 1.57 \times 10^5$)	1
JA10	ND[d]	ND
JA15	1.38×10^4 ($\pm 2.03 \times 10^3$)	0.016
JR1	1.33×10^7 ($\pm 2.69 \times 10^6$)	15.7

[a] Average *recA* copy number in 10 ng of total RNA from three biological replicates
[b] SD, standard deviation
[c] Fold change in average copy number from wild-type levels
[d] ND, Not detected

Table 2. *recA* transcript levels.

2.5 Characterization of the *recA* transcriptional unit

Analysis of the *B. burgdorferi* genome reveals two genes (BB0132 and BB0133) immediately upstream of *recA* (BB0131) that are oriented in the same direction (Fig. 5A). The reduced expression of *recA* in the JA15 complemented mutant may be the result of regulatory elements encoded outside of the 512 bp of upstream DNA amplified to generate the complementation construct pBB0131comp.2. It is also possible, given the organization of the flanking genes, that *recA* is co-transcribed with one or both of the upstream genes as part of

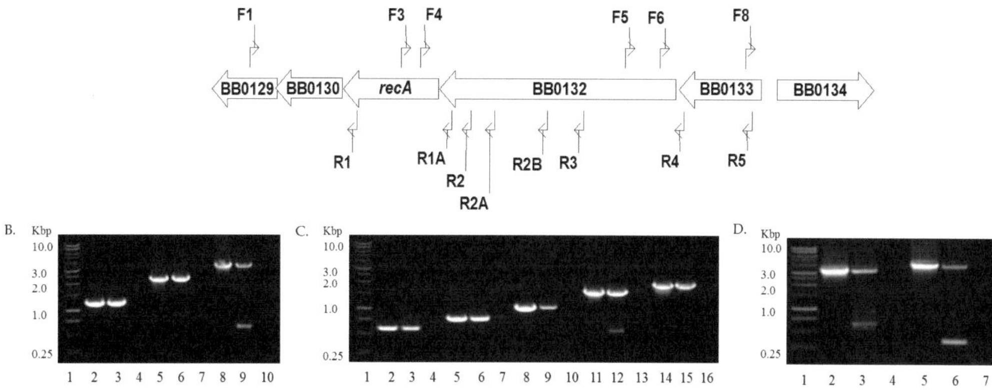

Fig. 5. Organization of *recA* and flanking genes. (A) Arrangement of the chromosomal region spanning genes BB0129 to BB0134 (7628 bp). Labeled arrows indicate the antisense and sense primers used for RT-PCR. (B) RT-PCR of B31-A RNA using a BB0129 antisense strand primer (F1) and sense strand primers R1 (lane 3), R1A (lanes 6) and R2B (lane 9). Positive control PCR reactions using B31-A genomic DNA as a template (lanes 2, 5 and 8) and no RT controls (lanes 4, 7 and 10) were also performed for each primer pair. (C) RT-PCR of B31-A RNA using a BB0131 (*recA*) antisense strand primer (F3) and sense strand primers R1A (lane 3), R2 (lane 6), R2A (lane 9), R2B (lane 12) and R3 (lane 15). Positive control PCR reactions using B31-A genomic DNA as a template (lanes 2, 5, 8, 11 and 14) and no RT controls (lanes 4, 7, 10, 13 and 16) were performed for each primer pair. (D) RT-PCR of B31-A RNA using a BB0131 (*recA*) antisense strand primer F3 with sense strand primers R4 (lane 3) and R5 (lane 6). Positive control PCR reactions using B31-A genomic DNA as a template (lanes 2 and 5) and no RT controls (lanes 4 and 7) were performed for each primer pair. A 1 kb ladder was used as a size standard (lane 1 of B, C and D).

an operon, and that the low level of expression observed in JA15 was due to a weak internal promoter. As previous studies have not evaluated the organization of the *recA* transcript in *B. burgdorferi*, we attempted to shed light on these questions by characterizing the *recA* transcriptional unit and identifying the *recA* promoter(s).

RT-PCR was used to determine if *recA* is co-transcribed with one or more of its neighboring genes (Fig. 5B-D). Antisense primers (F1 and F3; see Fig. 5) were used to generate cDNA from points originating in the downstream gene BB0129 and within the *recA* coding region. The cDNA was amplified in PCR reactions using the antisense primer and various sense primers to determine if mRNA transcripts spanned the junctions between adjacent genes. To determine if *recA* is co-transcribed with downstream genes, cDNA generated using primer F1 was PCR amplified using the same antisense primer and primers R1, R1A and R2B (Fig. 5B). All primer pairs produced products of the correct size when compared to positive controls, indicating the presence of an RNA transcript spanning genes BB0129-BB0132 and suggesting *recA* is co-transcribed with at least two downstream genes. In addition, the positive RT product obtained with primers F1 and R2B (lane 9; Fig. 5B) suggested that *recA* may be part of a larger operon encompassing one or both upstream genes, as the R2B primer was located 1.2 kb upstream of the *recA* translational start site. To confirm that *recA* is co-transcribed with BB0132, cDNA was generated using antisense primer F3 and PCR amplified using the same antisense primer and sense primers R1A, R2, R2A, R2B and R3

(Fig. 5C). An RT product of the correct size was obtained with all primer pairs when compared to the positive controls, confirming the results obtained with antisense primer F1 (Fig. 5B) and strongly suggesting that *recA* is co-transcribed with BB0132. To determine if BB0133 is also part of this transcriptional unit, cDNA generated with antisense primer F3 was PCR amplified using the same antisense primer and sense primers R4 and R5 (Fig. 5D). An RT product of the correct size was obtained with both primer pairs when compared to the positive controls, providing evidence that BB0133 is also part of this operon. Taken together, these RT results strongly suggest *recA* is co-transcribed with the upstream genes BB0132 and BB0133 and at least two downstream genes (BB0130 and BB0129).

2.6 5' RACE and promoter analysis

The RT results presented above strongly suggest that *recA* is co-transcribed with the upstream genes BB0132 and BB0133 (Fig. 5B-D); however, we did observe reduced expression of *recA* in our mutant complemented with the wild-type gene and 512 bp of upstream DNA (Table 2). Together, these results suggest two *recA* transcripts may exist, one beginning upstream of BB0133 and the other beginning within the 512 bp immediately upstream of the *recA* gene. Therefore, we used 5' RACE to identify the two *recA* transcritptional start sites, and compared the promoter regions upstream of the start sites to previously identified RpoD, RpoS and RpoN-dependent promoter sequences in *B. burgdorferi* (Studholme & Buck 2000; Caimano et al. 2007; Rhodes et al. 2009).

To identify the transcriptional start site immediately upstream of the *recA* gene, total RNA was extracted from B31-A cells cultured to late log phase (~2.0×10^7 cells ml^{-1}) in complete BSK-II and cDNA was generated using antisense primer F3 (Fig. 5A) located within the *recA* coding region. The cDNA was column purified and a homopolymeric A-tail was added using terminal transferase. PCR amplification of the A-tailed cDNA with nested gene specific primer F4 and an oligo dT-anchor primer resulted in a product of approximately 250 bp (lane 2; Fig. 6A). The DNA band was extracted from the gel and sequenced with primer F4, and the transcriptional start site was determined to be 44 or 45 bp upstream of the *recA* translational start (Fig. 6C). We attempted to clarify the start site using G-tailed cDNA, but were unable to obtain reliable sequence data for this PCR product due to mispriming of the oligo dC-anchor primer to three guanosines (underlined in Fig. 6C) located 29-31 bp upstream of the *recA* translational start site (data not shown). Based on the sequence data obtained from the A-tailed reaction we identified the putative -10 and -35 promoter regions immediately upstream of the *recA* gene. Comparison of these putative promoter regions with previously described *B. burgdorferi* promoter consensus sequences revealed similarity to the RpoD-dependent consensus promoter, as homology was observed in five of the six bases within the -35 region and seven of the eleven bases within the extended -10 region (Fig. 7).

To determine the transcriptional start site upstream of BB0133, total RNA was extracted from B31-A cells cultured to late log phase (~2.0×10^7 cells ml^{-1}) in complete BSK-II, and cDNA was generated using antisense primer F5 (Fig. 5A) located within BB0132. A homopolymeric A-tail was added and PCR of the A-tailed cDNA with nested gene specific primer F6 and the oligo dT-anchor primer resulted in a 1.2 kb product (Fig. 6B). The DNA band was gel extracted and sequenced with nested primer F8, and the transcriptional start site was determined to be 45 or 46 bp upstream of the BB0133 translational start site (Fig. 6D). Both G-tailed and C-tailed cDNA were used to try and resolve this ambiguity, but PCR

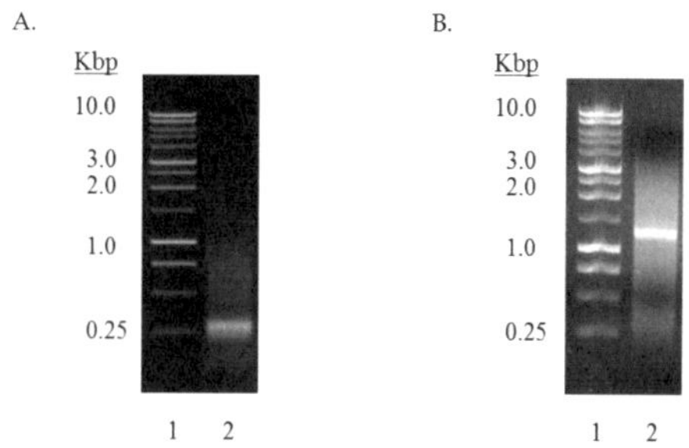

C. -10...TTTCCTAGCT AAATTTTATG GGTTCTATTT TTTTTACAAA ATATTTAAAA...-59 Upstream region of BB0131
...TTTCCTAGCT AAATTTTATG GGTTCTATTT TTTTTAAAAA AAAAAAAAAA... A-tailed 5′RACE product

D. -7...ACCATTTTAA ACAATATATA CAAACCCCCG TTACACTTTA TATAATTATA...-56 Upstream region of BB0133
...ACCATTTTAA ACAATATATA CAAACCCCCG TTACACTTTA AAAAAAAAAA... A-tailed 5′RACE product

Fig. 6. Identification of the transcriptional start sites of the *recA* transcript. 5′ RACE was used to determine the approximate transcriptional start sites of the *recA* transcript. A-tailed PCR products obtained using primer F4 (A; lane 2) or primer F6 (B; lane 2) with the oligo dT-anchor primer were separated by gel electrophoresis on a 1% TAE agarose gel. A 1 kb ladder was used as a size standard (lane 1). (C) DNA sequence of the dA-tailed 5′ RACE product obtained with primer F4 showing the approximate transcriptional start site (enlarged font). Underlined guanosines indicate site of mispriming with the oligo dC-anchor primer and dG-tailed 5′ RACE product. (D) DNA sequence of the dA-tailed 5′ RACE product obtained with primer F6 showing the approximate transcriptional start site (enlarged font).

Promoter	-35 Region		Extended -10 Region	Reference
Predicted *recA* promoters				
Upstream of *recA*	T T G T T A	-10-	T A A T T T T A A A T	This Study
Upstream of BB0133	T T G A C T	-11-	A A T G A T A T A A T	This Study
RpoD-dependent	T T g/a a/t a/c A		T A T G a/t T A T A a/c T	[8]
RpoS-dependent	T T G A a/t t/a		T G g/a g/a A T A t/a A T T	[26]
RpoS and RpoD-dependent	T T G A g/a N		t/a G a/c A c/g T A a/t a/g T T	[8]
RpoN-dependent	T G G C A C (-24 under GG)	N	N N N N T T G C W (-12 under GC)	[27]

Fig. 7. Identification of the putative *recA* promoters. Comparison of the putative *recA* promoters with the RpoD, RpoS and RpoN-dependent promoters in *B. burgdorferi*. Nucleotide positions in the predicted *recA* promoters that match the consensus RpoD-dependent promoter sequence are highlighted.

amplification with the nested primer F6 and the complementary-tailed anchor primers (C or G, respectively) did not produce a PCR product (data not shown). Therefore, we used the approximate transcriptional start site determined from the A-tailed cDNA to identify the putative -10 and -35 promoter regions. Comparison to *B. burgdorferi* consensus promoters suggests this operon is under the control of an RpoD-dependent promoter as homology was observed between five of the six bases within the -35 region and ten of eleven bases within the extended -10 region (Fig. 7).

2.7 Growth of the *recA* mutant in BSK-II without GlcNAc

Growth analysis of wild-type *B. burgdorferi* adapted to GlcNAc starvation suggests this organism undergoes a mutational event that allows growth to high cell densities in a single exponential phase in the absence of free GlcNAc (Figs. 2-4). Previous reports have demonstrated that DSBR proteins play a role in stress-induced mutations observed in other organisms (for reviews see (Galhardo et al. 2007; Hastings 2007)). Therefore, we evaluated the ability of a *recA* mutant in *B. burgdorferi* (JA10) to grow and adapt to GlcNAc starvation (Fig. 8). Late log phase *recA* mutant (JA10) cells cultured in complete BSK-II were diluted to 1.0×10^5 cells ml^{-1} in BSK-II lacking GlcNAc. Growth of the *recA* mutant prior to adaptation to GlcNAc starvation resulted in biphasic growth similar to wild-type cells that were not previously adapted to GlcNAc starvation (compare Fig. 8 open circles to Fig. 1A open circles). Similarly, when the *recA* mutant was diluted from the second exponential phase of a GlcNAc-starved culture (Fig. 8; 300 h) into the same medium biphasic growth was still observed (Fig. 8 open and closed triangles). This is in contrast to the single exponential phase typically observed in starvation-adapted wild-type cells that were cultured in the absence of GlcNAc (Fig. 1C).

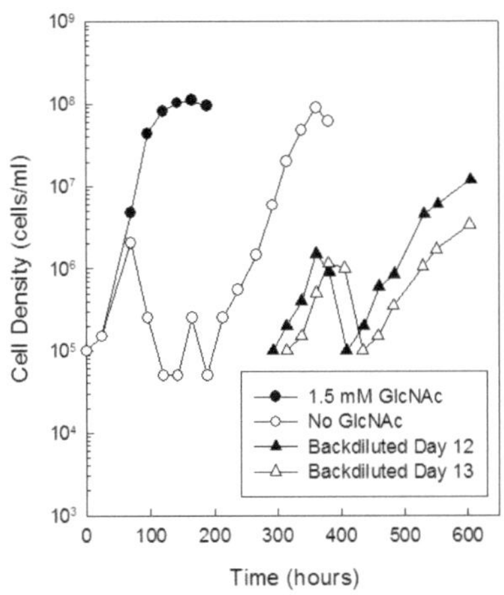

Fig. 8. Growth of JA10 (*recA* mutant) after adaptation to GlcNAc starvation. Growth of JA10 in BSK-II with and without 1.5 mM GlcNAc, and growth of JA10 cells after adaptation to GlcNAc starvation. Late log phase cells were diluted to 1.0×10^5 cells ml^{-1} in complete BSK-II (open circle) or BSK-II lacking GlcNAc (closed circle), and cells were enumerated daily by darkfield microscopy. Cells adapted to GlcNAc starvation were diluted (arrows) to 1.0×10^5 cells ml^{-1} at Day 12 (closed triangle) and Day 13 (open triangle) in BSK-II without GlcNAc, and growth was followed daily by darkfield microscopy.

Multiple growth experiments evaluating adaptation to GlcNAc starvation (i.e. dilution from the second exponential phase) were performed for each strain (Table 3). The growth experiment was repeated 15 times with *recA* mutant cells, and biphasic growth was observed each time cells were diluted from the second exponential phase of a culture starved for GlcNAc. This is in contrast to wild-type cells which exhibited biphasic growth only 3 times in 33 separate growth experiments, and reached high cell densities in a single exponential phase in 30 separate experiments.

Strain	Number of Growth Exp.[a]	Adapted[b]	Not Adapted[c]	Percent Adapted[d]
B31-A	33	30	3	91
JA10	15	0	15	0
JA15	17	5	12	29
JR1	13	3	10	23

[a] Number of independent growth experiments conducted in which cells were diluted from BSK-II lacking GlcNAc into the same medium

[b] Adapted - the number of times cells reached high cell density (1-2 × 10^7 cells ml^{-1}) in a single exponential phase

[c] Not Adapted - the number of times biphasic growth was observed

[d] Percent Adapted calculated as the number adapted (b) divided by the total number of experiments (a) multiplied by 100

Table 3. Adaptation to GlcNAc starvation.

To provide further evidence that RecA plays a role in the adaptation to GlcNAc starvation, we evaluated growth after GlcNAc starvation in the *recA* complemented mutants. Growth of the JA15 complemented mutant was followed in 17 separate experiments and single exponential phase growth to high cell densities in the absence of free GlcNAc was observed 5 times. Similarly, the JR1 complemented mutant was evaluated in 13 separate growth experiments and exhibited a single exponential phase in BSK-II lacking GlcNAc 3 times. Taken together, these results suggest RecA plays a role in adaptation to GlcNAc starvation and that the level of RecA expression may be important in the process.

3. Discussion

B. burgdorferi exhibits a unique biphasic growth pattern when cultured in the absence of free GlcNAc, with cells reaching optimal density in the second exponential phase. However, it had not been conclusively determined whether a physiologic or genetic adaptation mechanism is responsible for second exponential phase growth. This study was conducted to address this question as well as identify genes important to the process. We provide evidence that adaptation to GlcNAc starvation in *B. burgdorferi* is the result of a genetic event, and suggest a role for the homologous recombination protein RecA. In addition, we characterized the *recA* transcript and showed that transcription occurs from two different promoter sites.

In a previous report, Tilly et al (Tilly et al. 2001) suggested that the biphasic growth observed during *B. burgdorferi* cultivation in the absence of free GlcNAc was the result of a physiologic adaptation, as cells diluted from the second exponential phase into fresh medium lacking GlcNAc still exhibited biphasic growth. However, careful inspection of the growth curve from that study revealed that starvation-adapted cells grew nearly 10-fold higher in the first exponential phase after re-introduction into BSK-II lacking GlcNAc, than cells that were not previously exposed to the starvation condition (Tilly et al. 2001). To us, these results suggested that the adaptation that permitted second exponential phase growth was maintained by cells after passage in the same medium. We followed the growth of cells transferred from the second exponential phase into BSK-II lacking GlcNAc and found that wild-type cells grew to a high cell density in a single exponential phase (Fig. 1C) in 30 out of 33 independent growth experiments (Table 3). This indicated that adaptation to the starvation condition was retained by the cells in nearly all of the experiments. However, it was not clear whether the adaptation was physiologic or genetic, as the starvation-stress condition was never removed (i.e. cells were only transferred from the second exponential phase directly into media lacking GlcNAc). Since other microorganisms exhibit stress-induced mutagenesis in response to nutrient deprivation and other stresses (for reviews see (Finkel 2006; Galhardo et al. 2007; Hastings 2007)), we hypothesized that *B. burgdorferi* may use similar mechanisms to adapt to GlcNAc starvation.

To determine if adaptation to GlcNAc starvation was physiologic or genetic, starvation-adapted cells were serially passaged in complete BSK-II to relieve the starvation-stress, then re-introduced to the starvation-stress condition (i.e. BSK-II lacking GlcNAc). If adaptation was physiologic then cells should exhibit biphasic growth; however, we found that after as many as twelve serial passages in a complete medium, cells still reached high cell density in a single exponential phase when re-introduced to a medium lacking free GlcNAc (Fig. 2). In addition, starvation-adapted cells were plated on BSK-II agar after seven serial passages in complete BSK-II and the growth of ten clones was followed in BSK-II broth lacking GlcNAc. Eight of the ten clones grew to optimal cell densities in a single exponential phase (Fig. 3B). It is possible that the two clones exhibiting biphasic growth were never adapted and only able to persist due to the release of GlcNAc from sequestered sources by the cells that had undergone adaptation. It is also possible that these two clones were originally adapted to GlcNAc starvation, but during serial passage in complete media became de-adapted, exhibiting the original wild-type phenotype (discussed below). In any case, re-plating of one of the adapted clones (RR45) resulted in all ten clones growing to a high cell density in a single exponential phase (Fig. 4B). These results strongly suggest that *B. burgdorferi* undergoes stress-induced mutagenesis that allows cells to adapt to GlcNAc starvation.

As discussed above, stress-induced adaptive mutagenesis in the *E. coli* Lac assay results in either point mutants or amplification of the "leaky" *lac* region that relieves the stress and allows cells to utilize lactose (Cairns & Foster 1991). This adaptive mutagenesis occurs by a number of different pathways (Cairns & Foster 1991; Harris et al. 1994; Harris et al. 1999; McKenzie et al. 2000; McKenzie et al. 2001; Lombardo et al. 2004), three of which are present in *B. burgdorferi*: i) MMR, ii) RpoS starvation-stress-response and iii) homologous recombination by DSBR proteins. The gene or genes directly involved in the utilization of sequestered GlcNAc in the second exponential phase remain unknown; therefore, it is difficult to determine if the genetic adaptation observed in *B. burgdorferi* is the result of a point mutation, amplification or both. However, data collected under GlcNAc starvation conditions relating to these three pathways in *B. burgdorferi* may shed some light on this question.

MMR is a highly conserved process that repairs mismatched bases that arise during replication, increasing the fidelity of DNA replication 100 to 1000-fold (reviewed in (Kunkel& Erie 2005)). DNA mismatches are recognized by the MutS and MutL proteins, and the mismatched base is removed from the unmethylated strand by the endonuclease activity of MutH. A reduction in MMR activity during stationary phase has been described and is one mechanism by which mutation frequency is increased, possibly resulting in advantageous point mutations (not amplifications) that allow for adaptation to certain stresses (Feng et al. 1996; Harris et al. 1999). In addition, inactivation of MMR genes results in a mutator phenotype that has been observed in natural bacterial populations (LeClerc et al. 1996; Matic et al. 1997; Oliver et al. 2002). We evaluated our GlcNAc starvation-adapted clones for a mutation in *mutS* or *mutL* to determine if adaptation occurred due to inactivation of the MMR system. Genomic DNA was extracted from five starvation-adapted clones (Fig. 4, clones 1-5) and the *mutS* and *mutL* genes were sequenced along with 1 kb of flanking DNA on either side of the gene (data not shown). No mutations were observed in any of the clones, suggesting these clones have functional MMR systems and that adaptive mutation did not occur due to the absence of this important DNA repair pathway. It is unknown if MutS and MutL levels were reduced during GlcNAc starvation, but it may be of interest to determine these levels in future experiments.

The point mutants observed in the *E. coli* Lac assay require the presence of RpoS and the general stress response (Lombardo et al. 2004). It is unclear exactly how RpoS or components of the RpoS regulon regulate the formation of point mutations that confer the Lac+ phenotype, but it is known that RpoS promotes the use of the error-prone DNA polymerase DinB in DSBR (Ponder et al. 2005). As *B. burgdorferi* does not possess a DinB homologue or other error-prone DNA polymerases, it is unlikely this mechanism plays a role in adaptation of this spirochete to GlcNAc starvation. However, the RpoS regulon has also been shown to be necessary for adaptive amplification in the *E. coli* Lac assay (Lombardo et al. 2004), and previous studies conducted in our lab have demonstrated the importance of RpoS in GlcNAc starvation and biphasic growth (Rhodes et al. 2009). We reported a role for RpoS in the regulation of chitobiose utilization, and also demonstrated that an *rpoS* mutant was unable to initiate second exponential phase growth in the absence of GlcNAc until after 400 hours. In contrast, wild-type cells initiate a second exponential phase by 125 hours and reach optimal cell densities by 300 hours. It is possible the long delay observed in the *rpoS* mutant reflects the inability of these cells to amplify the gene(s) needed to obtain sequestered GlcNAc in the second exponential phase.

The DSBR protein RecA is also required for stress-induced point mutation and amplification in the *E. coli* Lac assay. With regard to point mutants, RecA most likely plays a role in increased mutagenesis through the up-regulation of the SOS response. As discussed above, *B. burgdorferi* does not possess the components for a functional SOS pathway, and so adaptive mutation in response to GlcNAc starvation by this mechanism is unlikely. However, homologous recombination and DSBR proteins such as RecA are also required for adaptation via amplification. Therefore, we evaluated the ability of a *recA* mutant to adapt to GlcNAc starvation by culturing cells in BSK-II without GlcNAc, and then diluting cells from the second exponential phase into the same medium. While the *recA* mutant exhibited biphasic growth similar to the wild type, these cells were unable to permanently adapt to GlcNAc starvation (Fig. 8) in any of the 15 independent experiments conducted (Table 3). These results suggest a role for RecA in the adaptation of wild-type cells to GlcNAc starvation, possibly through amplification of target gene(s) by homologous recombination.

Complementation of the *recA* mutant with two different complementation plasmids resulted in *recA* expression that was either 62.5-fold lower (JA15) or 15.7-fold higher (JR1) than wild-type expression (Table 2), and only partial restoration of the adaptive phenotype (Table 3). The partial restoration of the adaptive phenotype in the JA15 complemented mutant may be due to reduced levels of RecA protein resulting in less amplification of the target genes necessary for obtaining sequestered GlcNAc. While only partial restoration of the adaptive phenotype in the JR1 complemented mutant may be due to a deamplification of the repeated target gene(s) because of abnormally high levels of RecA. It has been observed in the *E. coli* Lac assay that *lac*-amplified clones (Lac^+) plated on rich medium containing a color indicator for β-galactosidase give rise to both white (Lac-) and sectored colonies (blue colonies with white sectors) due to deamplification of the repeated *lac* region, and that deamplification is mediated by RecA (Tlsty et al. 1984). This deamplification mechanism could also account for the two clones that exhibited biphasic growth in BSK-II lacking GlcNAc after repeated passage in complete BSK-II (Fig. 3B), and the three GlcNAc starvation experiments in wild-type cells that did not result in the adaptive phenotype (Table 3).

As a result of the reduced *recA* expression in our complemented mutant with the wild-type *recA* gene and 512 bp of upstream DNA (Table 2; JA15) we characterized the *recA* transcriptional unit (Fig. 5) and identified two putative promoters for this gene (Fig. 6 and 7). RT-PCR analysis confirmed that *recA* was co-transcribed with both upstream genes (BB0132 encoding the transcription elongation factor GreA; and BB0133 encoding a protein with a tetratricopeptide repeat domain) and at least two of the downstream genes (BB0130 encoding a conserved hypothetical protein; and BB0129 encoding an RNA-uridine isomerase). The combination of our RT-PCR data with our expression data from JA15 suggested the possibility of two promoters, one just upstream of the *recA* coding region and the other upstream of BB0133. We confirmed this using 5′ RACE (Fig. 6), and identified two putative promoters based on comparison to previously identified *B. burgdorferi* RpoD, RpoS and RpoN-dependent promoters (Fig. 7) (Studholme & Buck 2000; Caimano et al. 2007; Rhodes et al. 2009). The promoter identified upstream of BB0133 is nearly identical to the RpoD consensus promoter indicating constitutive expression under normal conditions, while the putative promoter immediately upstream of the *recA* coding region shows the most, but only limited, homology to the RpoD consensus sequence. In light of these results and the role *recA* plays in adaptation to GlcNAc starvation, it is interesting to speculate that the promoter immediately upstream of *recA* may be involved in the expression of this gene under specific cellular conditions or stresses.

4. Methods

4.1 Bacterial strains and culture conditions

The bacterial strains and plasmids used in this study are described in Table 4. Wild-type and mutant *B. burgdorferi* strains were routinely cultured in modified BSK-II (Barbour 1984) medium supplemented with 7% rabbit serum (Invitrogen, Corp.; Carlsbad, CA) and any necessary antibiotics. BSK-II was modified from the original recipe by replacing 10x CMRL-1066 with 10x Media 199 (Invitrogen). In addition, free GlcNAc was left out of BSK-II for certain growth experiments. For selection and maintenance of antibiotic resistance in *B. burgdorferi*, streptomycin, kanamycin and erythromycin were used at concentrations of 100 μg ml^{-1}, 340 μg ml^{-1} and 1 μg ml^{-1} respectively.

E. coli DH5α was used to maintain plasmids during cloning procedures and was cultured in lysogeny broth (LB; 1% tryptone, 0.5% yeast extract, 1% NaCl) with the appropriate antibiotic(s). Antibiotics were used at the following concentrations for *E. coli* DH5α: streptomycin, 100 μg ml^{-1}; kanamycin, 50 μg ml^{-1}; ampicillin, 200 μg ml^{-1}.

4.2 Growth curve analysis

For analysis of growth in liquid cultures, late-log phase cells (5.0×10^7 cells ml^{-1} to 1.0×10^8 cells ml^{-1}) were diluted to 1.0×10^5 cells ml^{-1} in BSK-II with or without GlcNAc. In general, 6-12 µl of culture was used to inoculate 6 ml of fresh culture medium; therefore, negligible amounts of free GlcNAc were transferred with the inoculum when analyzing growth in medium lacking GlcNAc. Cells were enumerated daily by darkfield microscopy using a Petroff-Hauser (Hauser Scientific; Horsham, PA) counting chamber. Specifically, 2.5 µl of liquid culture was transferred to the counting chamber, and cells in all 25 squares were counted. Cells were diluted 1:10 in BSK-II prior to counting when the culture density was greater than 1.0×10^7 cells ml^{-1}. All growth experiments were carried out at 33°C in the presence of 3% CO_2. Unless otherwise stated, each growth curve presented in this study is representative of at least three independent trials, as growth data could not be pooled due to the length of experiments and the different times at which bacteria were enumerated.

4.3 Construction of a *recA* mutant in *B. burgdorferi*

The construct used to generate a *recA* (BB0131) mutation in the B31-A background was created as follows: i) A 2.1 kb fragment of the 3′ end of BB0131 and flanking DNA was PCR amplified with engineered restriction sites using primers (Table 5) 5′ BB0131 mutF1 (KpnI) and 5′ BB0131 mutR2 (XbaI); ii) the PCR fragment was TA cloned into pCR2.1 (Invitrogen) to generate plasmid pBB0131.1; iii) plasmids pBB0131.1 and pKFSS1 (Frank et al. 2003) (a *B. burgdorferi* shuttle vector conferring streptomycin resistance; Table 4) were digested with KpnI and XbaI and separated by gel electrophoresis; iv) the 2.1 kb band from pBB0131.1 was gel extracted and cloned into the gel extracted pKFSS1 fragment to generate pBB0131.2; v) the 2.1 kb fragment and flanking streptomycin resistance gene were PCR amplified from pBB0131.2 using primers 5′ BB0131 mutF1 (KpnI) and pKFSS1 R1; vi) the 3.6 kb amplicon was TA cloned into pGEM T-Easy (Promega, Corp.; Madison, WI) to generate pBB0131.3A or B (based on the orientation of the PCR product insertion); vii) plasmid pBB0131.3B was identified by restriction digest in which the 3′ end of the streptomycin resistance gene was adjacent to the XmaI site in the pGEM T-Easy vector; viii) the 5′ end of BB0131 and flanking DNA (1.8 kb) was PCR amplified with engineered restriction sites using primers 3′ BB0131 mutF1 (XmaI) and 3′ BB0131 mutR1 (SacII) and TA cloned into pCR2.1 to generate pBB0131.4; ix) plasmids pBB0131.3B and pBB0131.4 were digested with XmaI and SacII and separated by gel electrophoresis; x) the 1.8 kb fragment from pBB0131.4 was gel extracted and cloned into the gel extracted fragment from pBB0131.3B to generate the final construct pBB0131.5. All plasmids were confirmed by restriction digest and DNA sequencing. In summary, 877 of the 1098 bp constituting the *recA* coding region were deleted and replaced with the streptomycin resistance gene transcribed in the opposite orientation and under the control of the constitutive *B. burgdorferi flgB* promoter. Plasmid pBB0131.5 was confirmed by PCR using primers flanking the antibiotic insertion site (BB0131 mut confirm F1 and 5′ recA SalI) that resulted in a 1.7 kb fragment (Fig. 9, lane 3) compared to a 1.2 kb fragment generated with the wild-type genomic DNA as a template (Fig. 9, lane 2).

To generate the *recA* deletion mutant, competent B31-A cells were prepared and transformed with 15 µg of pBB0131.5 as previously described (Samuels et al. 1994). Briefly, transformed cells were resuspended in 10 ml of complete BSK-II and allowed to recover overnight at 33°C. The transformation reaction was plated in solid BSK-II medium containing 100 μg ml^{-1} streptomycin to select for the allelic exchange event. Streptomycin resistant colonies were screened by PCR using primers that flanked the insertion site. One clone (JA10) was chosen for further experimentation and PCR of the genomic DNA from this strain with the primers BB0131 mut confirm F1 and 5′ recA SalI demonstrated the presence of the mutant *recA* allele (Fig. 9, lane 5). In addition, the insertion was confirmed by DNA sequencing of the PCR product.

Strain or Plasmid	Genotype and Description	Reference
Strains		
B . burgdorferi		
B31-A	High passage non-infectious wild-type	(Elias et al. 2000)
RR45	GlcNAc starvation adapted clone	This study
JA10	Str^R; B31-A *recA* mutant	This study
JA15	Str^R Kan^R; JA10 complemented with pBB0131comp.2	This study
JR1	Str^R Kan^R; JA10 complemented with precA.2	This study
E. coli		
DH5α	*supE*44 F^- Δ*lac*U169 (ϕ80*lacZ* ΔM15) *hsdR*17 *relA*1 *endA*1 *gyrA*96 *thi*-1 *relA*1	(Hanahan 1983)
Plasmids		
pKFSS1	Str^R; *B. burgdorferi* shuttle vector, cp9 based	(Frank et al. 2003)
pBSV2	Kan^R; *B. burgdorferi* shuttle vector, cp9 based	(Stewart et al. 2001)
pCE320	Kan^R Zeo^R; *B. burgdorferi* shuttle vector, cp32 based	(Eggers et al. 2002)
ErmC/pCE320	Kan^R Zeo^R, Erm^R; *B. burgdorferi* shuttle vector, cp32 based	This study
pBB0450.1	Erm^R; *ermC*::BB0450	(Rhodes et al. 2009)
pBB0131.5	Str^R; *aadA*::BB0131 (*recA*)	This study
pBB0131comp.2	Kan^R; BB0131 complementation construct - *recA* with 512 bp of upstream DNA	This study
pRecA.3	Kan^R; BB0131 complementation construct –*recA* fused to constitutive *flaB* promoter	This study

Table 4. Strains and plasmids used in this study.

Primer Name	Sequence (5′→ 3′)
5′ BB0131 mutF1 (KpnI)	GCTAGGGTACCTGCTTATATCGCCTCAAAGCTCG
5′ BB0131 mutR2 (XbaI)	GCTAGTCTAGACTTAGCAAAGAAGTAGAACTTGC
pKFSS1 R1	TGATGAACAGGGTCACGTCGTC
3′ BB0131 mutF1 (XmaI)	GCTAGCCCGGGGCTTTTTCTATTTGAACTCTTGCAAGC
3′ BB0131 mutR1 (SacII)	GCTAGCCGCGGTATGGCCATGTCGGCTTTATCTCC
BB0131 mut confirm F1	CAAGGCTGATAGAGTAACTACCCA
BB0131 comp F1 (KpnI)	GCTAGGGTACCCAAGGCTGATAGAGTAACTACCCA
BB0131 comp R1 (XbaI)	GCTAGTCTAGATGCAGGCGAGAGAATGGAAATTGG
PflaB F1 (SalI)	GTCGACATATCATTCCTCCATGATAAAATTT
PflaB R1 (NotI)	GCGGCCGCTGTCTGTCGCCTCTTGTGG
5′ recA (SalI)	GTCGACATGTCAAAGTTAAAGGAAAAAAGAGAAAAAGC
BbrecA F1	CAAGGCTGATAGAGTAACTACCCA
ErmC F1	GGTTCCATAATATGTTCTCCCTTTCTCAG
ErmC R1	CCCAACGCTCGAATTTAAAGACCC
recA operon F1	CACGCTCTTTAAATAAGGGCTGAACC
recA operon F3	AATCTCAAGAGCTTGCTCTCCGGT
recA operon F4	CCAATGCCGAGAGCCTCATCTAAT
recA operon F5	TGGCCCATACTTCTCTGATTCCTG
recA operon F6	ACGTCCTTTAAATGCCTGCCAC
recA operon F8	CAAGGCTTTCAACTTGACCATTCCA
recA operon R1	CAGGCTCATGGTATTCATTGGGAG
recA operon R1A	TACTTGGGCCTTGGGAATCAAACC
recA operon R2	AAAGCTCGTGAACTTGGTGA
recA operon R2A	ATCGGTCTTAGAGGTCGTGAGAGA
recA operon R2B	AGGATTTGCATATTGAAGAAGAGATGC
recA operon R3	TATGGCCATGTCGGCTTTATCTCC
recA operon R4	GAAGATAGAGCACGTATTGATGAG
recA operon R5	CCGAAGAGGCTCATTCTCTTGA
oligo dT-anchor primer	GACCACGCGTATCGATGTCGACTTTTTTTTTTTTTTTTV
BB0131 F1	ACATCATCGCTTGAGCCCGATCTA
BB0131 R1	ACCACTACCGGTGGGAATGCTTTA

Table 5. Oligonucleotide primers used in this study

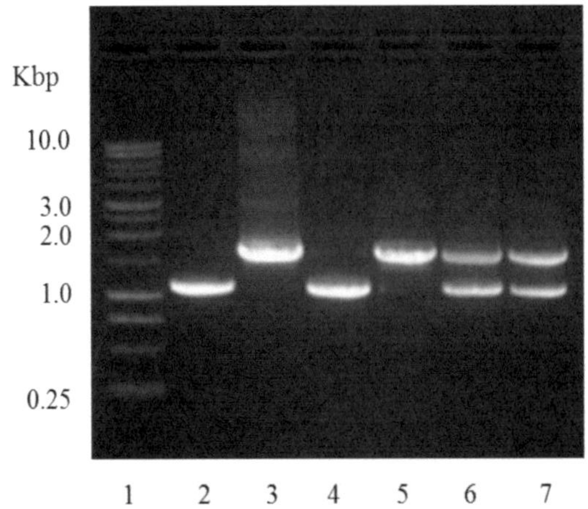

Fig. 9. PCR confirmation of the *recA* mutant and complemented mutant strains. PCR confirmation of JA10 (*recA* deletion/insertion mutant), JA15 (JA10 complemented with pBB0131comp.2) and JR1 (JA10 complemented with pRecA.3) using primers BB0131 mut confirm F1 and 5′ recA SalI which flank the insertion site. The larger PCR product is 1.7 kb (upper arrow) and contains the streptomycin resistance gene within *recA*. The smaller PCR product is 1.2 kb (lower arrow) and represents the wild-type *recA* gene. PCR reactions using the following templates were separated by electrophoresis: lane 1 - 1 kb ladder (Promega), lane 2 - B31-A genomic DNA, lane 3 - pBB0131.5 (*recA* mutation construct), lane 4 - pRecA.3 (complementation plasmid for JR1), lane 5 - JA10 genomic DNA (*recA* mutant), lane 6 - JA15 genomic DNA (JA10 complemented with pBB0131comp.2) and lane 7 - JR1 genomic DNA (JA10 complemented with pRecA.3).

4.4 Complementation of the *recA* mutant

Two approaches were used to complement the *recA* mutation in JA10. First, the *recA* gene and 512 bp of upstream DNA were PCR amplified using primers BB0131 comp F1 (KpnI) and BB0131 comp R1 (XbaI), and the 1.6 kb fragment was TA cloned into pCR2.1 to generate pBB0131comp.1. Plasmids pBB0131comp.1 and pBSV2 (Stewart et al. 2001) (*E. coli-B. burgdorferi* shuttle conferring kanamycin resistance), were digested with KpnI and XbaI and separated by gel electrophoresis. The 1.6 kb fragment from pBB0131comp.1 was gel extracted and ligated with the gel extracted fragment from pBSV2 to generate pBB0131comp.2. Fifteen micrograms of pBB0131comp.2 was transformed into competent JA10 cells and transformants were selected by plating on solid BSK-II medium containing 100 μg ml^{-1} streptomycin and 340 μg ml^{-1} kanamycin. Clones were screened by PCR using primers BB0131 mut confirm F1 and 5′ recA SalI. One clone, designated JA15, was selected for further experimentation and the presence of both the mutant and wild-type *recA* alleles was confirmed by PCR using 50 ng of genomic DNA as template (Fig. 9; lane 6).

We also generated a complementation construct in which we fused the wild-type *recA* gene to the constitutive *B. burgdorferi flaB* promoter. The *flaB* promoter was PCR amplified from B31-A genomic DNA using primers PflaB F1 (SalI) and PflaB R1 (NotI), and cloned into pCR2.1 to generate pPflaB. The *recA* coding region was PCR amplified from B31-A genomic DNA using primers 5′ recA (SalI) and BbrecA F1, and cloned into pCR2.1 to generate pRecA.1. Plasmids pPflaB and pRecA.1 were digested with SalI and NotI and separated by gel electrophoresis. The 360 bp product from pPflaB was gel extracted and ligated into the gel extracted fragment of pRecA.1 to generate pRecA.2. The *flaB* promoter-*recA* fusion was removed from pRecA.2 by digestion with KpnI and XbaI (sites in pCR2.1 flanking the TA insertion site), separated by gel electrophoresis, gel extracted and cloned into like sites in pCE320 (Eggers et al. 2002) (a *B. burgdorferi* shuttle vector with a circular plasmid 32 (cp32) origin for replication that confers kanamycin resistance) to generate pRecA.3. The complementation construct pRecA.3 was concentrated and transformed into JA10 as described above. Transformants were screened by PCR using primers BB0131 mut confirm F1 and 5′ recA SalI, and one clone was designated JR1 and used for further experiments. PCR using 50 ng of JR1 genomic DNA resulted in amplification of both wild-type and mutant *recA* alleles (Fig. 9; lane 7).

4.5 Homologous recombination assay

A homologous recombination assay similar to that described previously by Liveris *et al* (Liveris et al. 2008) was used to determine transformation and recombination frequencies for the wild-type, *recA* mutant and *recA* complemented mutant strains. To determine transformation frequency we generated plasmid ErmC/pCE320 in which the pCE320 shuttle vector was modified to confer erythromycin resistance. Specifically, primers ErmC F1 and ErmC R1 were used to amplify the erythromycin resistance gene and its corresponding promoter from plasmid pBB0450.1, which was then TA cloned into pCR2.1 to generate pCR2.1/ErmC. Plasmid pCR2.1/ErmC was digested with BamHI and NotI, separated by gel electrophoresis, and the fragment containing *ermC* was gel extracted and cloned into like sites in pCE320 to generate ErmC/pCE320. Plasmid ErmC/pCE320 was concentrated to >1 μg μl^{-1} and cells were electroporated with 15 μg of plasmid as previously described (Samuels et al. 1994). After recovery overnight in BSK-II, transformants were selected on solid BSK-II containing 1 μg ml^{-1} erythromycin and transformation frequency was calculated by dividing the number of transformant colonies obtained by the total number of cells plated (CFU) as determined by dilution and plating without antibiotic selection. The presence of ErmC/pCE320 was confirmed in at least ten erythromycin resistant colonies from each experiment by colony PCR with primers specific for *ermC*.

The ability of *recA* expressing and non-expressing strains to mediate allelic exchange was determined by calculating the recombination frequency following electroporation with plasmid pBB0450.1 (*rpoN::ermC* with flanking DNA) (Rhodes et al. 2009). Transformation and plating with pBB0450.1 was carried out as described above for ErmC/pCE320 and recombinants were selected on solid BSK-II containing 1 μg ml^{-1} erythromycin. Recombination frequency was calculated by dividing the number of erythromycin resistant colonies by the total number of cells plated (CFU) as determined by dilution and plating without selection. Allelic exchange was confirmed in at least ten erythromycin resistant colonies from each experiment by colony PCR with primers flanking the insertion site in *rpoN*.

4.6 RNA extraction

RNA was extracted from wild-type cells (B31-A) for use in RT-PCR and qRT-PCR experiments. Briefly, cells were harvested during mid to late log phase (1.0 to 5.0×10^7 cells ml^{-1}) by centrifugation (10,000 × *g*, 12 min, 4°C). Pellets were resuspended in 500 μl of cold BSK-II and transferred to a 2 ml microcentrifuge tube. One milliliter of Bacteria RNAProtect

(Qiagen; Valencia, CA) was added, mixed by vortexing and incubated for 5 min at room temperature. Cells were collected by centrifugation at 5,000 × *g* for 10 min, the supernatant was decanted and pellets were stored at -80°C for up to 4 weeks prior to RNA extraction. RNA was extracted using the RNeasy Mini kit (Qiagen) according to the manufacturer's instructions and treated with RQ1 RNase-free DNase (Promega, Corp.) and RNasin (Promega, Corp.) to remove any contaminating genomic DNA. RNA was purified using the RNeasy Mini kit and following the RNA Clean-up protocol supplied by the manufacturer. RNA concentration (OD_{260}) and purity ($OD_{260/280}$) were determined by UV spectroscopy using the Nanodrop ND-1000 (Nanodrop products of Thermo Fisher Scientific; Wilmington, DE) and RNA integrity was verified by visualizing the intensity of the 16S and 23S rRNA bands on a 1% agarose gel. RNA was concentrated to greater that 1 $\mu g\ \mu l^{-1}$ by isopropanol precipitation and stored at -80°C.

4.7 Quantitative RT-PCR (qRT-PCR) to determine *recA* expression

qRT-PCR was performed using the Mx3005P Multiplex Quantitative PCR System in conjunction with the Brilliant SYBR Green Single-Step qRT-PCR Master Mix kit (Stratagene; La Jolla, CA) according to the manufacturer's instructions. Briefly, a standard curve (10^1 to 10^7 copies per reaction) was prepared using a purified *recA* PCR product that was generated from B31-A genomic DNA using primers BB0131 F1 and BB0131 R1. Reactions (25 μl) containing 10 ng of total RNA extracted from mid-log phase cells (~1.0×10^7 cells ml^{-1}) were run under the following conditions: 1 cycle of 50°C for 30 min and 95°C for 15 min, followed by 40 cycles of 95°C for 30 s and 58°C for 30 s. Fluorescence was measured at the end of the 58°C step every cycle. Triplicate samples for each experiment were averaged, and the average and standard deviations were calculated for three independent experiments. All qRT-PCR experiments included both no-reverse transcriptase (RT) and no-template controls. The *recA* copy number for each sample was calculated using the MxPro (Stratagene) data analysis software and the *recA* standard curve described above. Copy number in each sample was normalized based on the total RNA input (10 ng per reaction) and the fold difference in *recA* copy number was determined by comparing the expression in the *recA* mutant and complemented mutant strains to the expression in the wild-type strain.

4.8 RT-PCR to determine the *recA* transcriptional unit

RT-PCR was used to determine the organization of the *recA* transcriptional unit. Complementary DNA (cDNA) was generated from B31-A RNA using the SuperScript® First Strand Synthesis for RT-PCR kit (Invitrogen, Corp.) according to the manufacturer's instructions. Briefly, 0.5 μg of RNA was reverse transcribed with SuperScript II RT enzyme at 42°C for one hour using gene specific primers recA operon F1 or F3. The RT enzyme was heat inactivated and RNA was degraded from the RNA-cDNA hybrid using RNaseH. To confirm there was no genomic DNA contamination a separate no RT reaction was run in conjunction with each RT reaction. For PCR, antisense primers used to generate the cDNA were used in various combinations with the sense primers recA operon R1, R1A, R2, R2A, R2B, R3, R4 or R5. Three reactions were prepared for each primer set and the following templates were added: i) 50 ng of B31-A genomic DNA, ii) 2 μl of the appropriate cDNA reaction, and iii) 2 μl of the appropriate no RT control reaction. Templates were amplified using TaKaRa ExTaq (Fisher Scientific; Pittsburgh, PA) and the following thermal cycle: i) initial denaturation for 10 min at 95°C, ii) 35 cycles of 95°C for 30 sec, 58°C for 30 sec and 72°C for 1 to 4 min (depending on the size of the expected product), and iii) final extension at 72°C for 10 min. PCR products were separated on a 1% agarose gel and visualized using ethidium bromide.

4.9 5' Rapid Amplification of cDNA Ends (RACE) and promoter analysis

The approximate *recA* transcriptional start sites were determined using the 2nd Generation 5'/3' RACE Kit (Roche Applied Science; Mannheim, Germany) according to the manufacturer's instructions. Briefly, two first-strand cDNA synthesis reactions were performed with 1 µg of total RNA and antisense primers recA operon F3 and recA operon F5 to determine the transcritptional start sites immediately upstream of BB0131 (*recA*) and BB0133. The two cDNA reactions were purified using the High Pure PCR Product Purification Kit (Roche Applied Science). The purified cDNAs were divided into two reaction tubes and a homopolymeric A or G-tail was added to the 3' end using recombinant terminal deoxynucleotidyl transferase and dATP or dGTP. A PCR product was amplified from each tailed cDNA using the appropriate anchor primer (oligo dT-AP or oligo dC-AP) and a nested gene specific primer. Nested primer recA operon F4 was used to amplify tailed cDNA generated with recA operon F3, and nested primer recA operon F6 was used to amplify tailed cDNA generated with recA operon F5. The PCR products were subjected to electrophoresis and the bands were gel extracted using the QIAquick PCR Purification Kit (Qiagen). The sequence of the purified PCR products were determined using either recA operon F4 or recA operon F8 and aligned to the upstream sequence of *recA* or BB0133 to determine the transcriptional start sites. Promoter analysis was carried out by visual inspection and comparison of the region upstream of the approximate transcriptional start sites with previously described RpoD, RpoS and RpoN-dependent promoter sequences in *B. burgdorferi*.

4.10 Nucleotide sequencing and computer analysis

Nucleic acid sequencing was performed by the Rhode Island Genomics and Sequencing Center using a 3130xl Genetic Analyzer (Applied Biosystems; Forest City, CA). Sequencing reactions were prepared using the BigDye® Terminator v3.0 Cycle Sequencing Kit. Sequences were analyzed using DNASTAR Lasergene software (DNASTAR, Inc.; Madison, WI) and Vector NTI (Invitrogen, Corp.).

5. Conclusions

In this study we demonstrate that *B. burgdorferi* undergoes a genetic adaptation during GlcNAc starvation that allows cells to grow to a high cell density when re-introduced to the starvation condition. We also show that *recA* mutant cells do not respond to GlcNAc starvation the same as wild-type cells, suggesting a role for RecA in this process. Finally, we characterize the *recA* transcriptional unit and provide evidence that this gene is controlled transcriptionally from two separate promoters.

6. Acknowledgments

We thank P. Rosa and J. Radolf for providing strains and plasmids. This research is based in part upon work conducted using the Rhode Island Genomics and Sequencing Center, which is supported in part by the National Science Foundation under EPSCoR Grant No. 0554548. This work was supported by NIH grant 5 R01AI03723010 awarded to DRN.

7. References

Barbour, A. G. (1984). "Isolation and cultivation of Lyme disease spirochetes." *The Yale Journal of Biology and Medicine* 57(4): 521-5.

Caimano, M. J., R. Iyer, C. H. Eggers, C. Gonzalez, E. A. Morton, M. A. Gilbert, I. Schwartz & J. D. Radolf (2007). "Analysis of the RpoS regulon in *Borrelia burgdorferi* in response to mammalian host signals provides insight into RpoS function during the enzootic cycle." *Molecular Microbiology* 65(5): 1193-1217.

Cairns, J. & P. L. Foster (1991). "Adaptive Reversion of a Frameshift Mutation in *Escherichia coli*." *Genetics* 128(4): 695-701.

Cox, M. M. (2007). "Regulation of Bacterial RecA Protein Function." *Critical Reviews in Biochemistry and Molecular Biology* 42(1): 41-63.

Das, R., Hegyi H, Gerstein M (2000). "Genome analyses of spirochetes: a study of the protein structures, functions and metabolic pathways in *Treponema pallidum* and *Borrelia burgdorferi*." *Journal of Molecular Microbiology and Biotechnololgy* 2(4): 387-392.

Eggers, C. H., M. J. Caimano, M. L. Clawson, W. G. Miller, D. S. Samuels & J. D. Radolf (2002). "Identification of loci critical for replication and compatibility of a *Borrelia burgdorferi* cp32 plasmid and use of a cp32-based shuttle vector for the expression of fluorescent reporters in the Lyme disease spirochaete." *Molecular Microbiology* 43(2): 281-295.

Elias, A. F., J. L. Bono, J. A. Carroll, P. Stewart, K. Tilly & P. Rosa (2000). "Altered stationary-phase response in a *Borrelia burgdorferi rpoS* mutant." *Journal of Bacteriology* 182(10): 2909-2918.

Feng, G., H. Tsui & M. Winkler (1996). "Depletion of the cellular amounts of the MutS and MutH methyl-directed mismatch repair proteins in stationary-phase *Escherichia coli* K-12 cells." *Journal of Bacteriology* 178(8): 2388-2396.

Finkel, S. E. (2006). "Long-term survival during stationary phase: evolution and the GASP phenotype." *Nature Reviews Microbiology* 4(2): 113-120.

Foster, P. L. & J. M. Trimarchi (1994). "Adaptive reversion of a frameshift mutation in *Escherichia coli* by simple base deletions in homopolymeric runs." *Science* 265(5170): 407-409.

Frank, K. L., S. F. Bundle, M. E. Kresge, C. H. Eggers & D. S. Samuels (2003). "*aadA* confers streptomycin resistance in *Borrelia burgdorferi*." *Journal of Bacteriology* 185(22): 6723-6727.

Galhardo, R. S., P. J. Hastings & S. M. Rosenberg (2007). "Mutation as a stress response and the regulation of evolvability." *Critical Reviews in Biochemistry and Molecular Biology* 42(5): 399-435.

Hanahan, D. (1983). "Studies on transformation of *Escherichia coli* with plasmids." *Journal of Molecular Biology* 166: 557-580.

Harris, R. S., G. Feng, K. J. Ross, R. Sidhu, C. Thulin, S. Longerich, S. K. Szigety, P. J. Hastings, M. E. Winkler & S. M. Rosenberg (1999). "Mismatch repair is diminished during stationary-phase mutation." *Mutation Research* 437(1): 51-60.

Harris, R. S., S. Longerich & S. M. Rosenberg (1994). "Recombination in adaptive mutation." *Science* 264(5156): 258-260.

Hastings, P. J. (2007). "Adaptive amplification." *Critical Reviews in Biochemistry and Molecular Biology* 42(4): 271-283.

Hastings, P. J., H. J. Bull, J. R. Klump & S. M. Rosenberg (2000). "Adaptive amplification: an inducible chromosomal instability mechanism." *Cell* 103(5): 723-731.

He, A. S., P. R. Rohatgi, M. N. Hersh & S. M. Rosenberg (2006). "Roles of *E. coli* double-strand-break-repair proteins in stress-induced mutation." *DNA Repair* 5(2): 258-273.

Kugelberg, E., E. Kofoid, A. B. Reams, D. I. Andersson & J. R. Roth (2006). "Multiple pathways of selected gene amplification during adaptive mutation." *Proceedings of the National Academy of Sciences of the United States of America* 103(46): 17319-17324.

Kunkel, T. A. & D. A. Erie (2005). "DNA mismatch repair." *Annual Review of Biochemistry* 74(1): 681-710.

Kurtenbach, K., K. Hanincova, J. I. Tsao, G. Margos, D. Fish & N. H. Ogden (2006). "Fundamental processes in the evolutionary ecology of Lyme borreliosis." *Nature Reviews Microbiology* 4(9): 660-669.

LeClerc, J. E., B. Li, W. L. Payne & T. A. Cebula (1996). "High mutation frequencies among *Escherichia coli* and *Salmonella* pathogens." *Science* 274(5290): 1208-1211.

Liveris, D., V. Mulay, S. Sandigursky & I. Schwartz (2008). "*Borrelia burgdorferi vlsE* antigenic variation is not mediated by RecA." *Infection and Immunity* 76(9): 4009-4018.

Liveris, D., V. Mulay & I. Schwartz (2004). "Functional properties of *Borrelia burgdorferi recA*." *Journal of Bacteriology* 186(8): 2275-2280.

Lombardo, M.-J., I. Aponyi & S. M. Rosenberg (2004). "General stress response regulator RpoS in adaptive mutation and amplification in *Escherichia coli*." *Genetics* 166(2): 669-680.

Matic, I., M. Radman, F. Taddei, B. Picard, C. Doit, E. Bingen, E. Denamur, J. Elion, J. E. LeClerc & T. A. Cebula (1997). "Highly variable mutation rates in commensal and pathogenic *Escherichia coli*." *Science* 277(5333): 1833-1834.

McKenzie, G. J., R. S. Harris, P. L. Lee & S. M. Rosenberg (2000). "The SOS response regulates adaptive mutation." *Proceedings of the National Academy of Sciences of the United States of America* 97(12): 6646-6651.

McKenzie, G. J., P. L. Lee, M.-J. Lombardo, P. J. Hastings & S. M. Rosenberg (2001). "SOS mutator DNA polymerase IV functions in adaptive mutation and not adaptive amplification." *Molecular Cell* 7(3): 571-579.

Oliver, A., F. Baquero & J. Blázquez (2002). "The mismatch repair system *mutS, mutL* and *uvrD* genes in *Pseudomonas aeruginosa*: molecular characterization of naturally occurring mutants." *Molecular Microbiology* 43(6): 1641-1650.

Ponder, R. G., N. C. Fonville & S. M. Rosenberg (2005). "A switch from high-fidelity to error-prone DNA double-strand break repair underlies stress-induced mutation." *Molecular Cell* 19(6): 791-804.

Powell, S. C. & R. M. Wartell (2001). "Different characteristics distinguish early versus late arising adaptive mutations in *Escherichia coli* FC40." *Mutation Research: Fundamental and Molecular Mechanisms of Mutagenesis* 473(2): 219-228.

Putteet-Driver, A. D., J. Zhong & A. G. Barbour (2004). "Transgenic expression of RecA of the spirochetes *Borrelia burgdorferi* and *Borrelia hermsii* in *Escherichia coli* revealed differences in DNA repair and recombination phenotypes." *Journal of Bacteriology* 186(8): 2266-2274.

Rhodes, R., W. Coy & D. Nelson (2009). "Chitobiose utilization in *Borrelia burgdorferi* is dually regulated by RpoD and RpoS." *BMC Microbiology* 9(1): 108.

Rhodes, R. G., J. A. Atoyan & D. R. Nelson (2010). "The chitobiose transporter, *chbC*, is required for chitin utilization in *Borrelia burgdorferi*." *BMC Microbiology* 10: 21.

Rosenberg, S. M., S. Longerich, P. Gee & R. S. Harris (1994). "Adaptive mutation by deletions in small mononucleotide repeats." *Science* 265(5170): 405-407.

Saier MH, J., Paulsen IT (2000). "Whole genome analyses of transporters in spirochetes: *Borrelia burgdorferi* and *Treponema pallidum*." *Journal of Molecular Microbiology and Biotechnology* 2(4): 393-9.

Samuels, D. S., K. E. Mach & C. F. Garon (1994). "Genetic transformation of the Lyme disease agent *Borrelia burgdorferi* with coumarin-resistant *gyrB*." *Journal of Bacteriology* 176(19): 6045-9.

Slack, A., P. C. Thornton, D. B. Magner, S. M. Rosenberg & P. J. Hastings (2006). "On the mechanism of gene amplification induced under stress in *Escherichia coli*." *Public Library of Science: Genetics* 2(4): e48.

Steere, A. C. (2001). "Lyme Disease." *The New England Journal of Medicine* 345(2): 115-125.

Steere, A. C., J. Coburn & L. Glickstein (2004). "The emergence of Lyme disease." *Journal of Clinical Investigation* 113(8): 1093-1101.

Stewart, P. E., R. Thalken, J. L. Bono & P. Rosa (2001). "Isolation of a circular plasmid region sufficient for autonomous replication and transformation of infectious *Borrelia burgdorferi*." *Molecular Microbiology* 39(3): 714-721.

Studholme, D. J. & M. Buck (2000). "The biology of enhancer-dependent transcriptional regulation in bacteria: insights from genome sequences." *Federation of European Microbiological Societies: Microbiology Letters* 186(1): 1-9.

Tilly, K., A. F. Elias, J. Errett, E. Fischer, R. Iyer, I. Schwartz, J. L. Bono & P. Rosa (2001). "Genetics and regulation of chitobiose utilization in *Borrelia burgdorferi*." *Journal of Bacteriology* 183(19): 5544-5553.

Tlsty, T. D., A. M. Albertini & J. H. Miller (1984). "Gene amplification in the *lac* region of *E. coli*." *Science* 37(1): 217-224.

7

Porins in the Genus *Borrelia*

Iván Bárcena-Uribarri[1], Marcus Thein[2], Mari Bonde[3], Sven Bergström[3] and Roland Benz[1,2]
[1]*Jacobs University Bremen*
[2]*University of Wuerzburg*
[3]*University of Umea*
[1,2]*Germany*
[3]*Sweden*

1. Introduction

1.1 The cell envelope of *Borrelia* compared to other gram-negative bacteria

Borreliae belong to the spirochete phylum, an ancient evolutionary branch only remotely related to Gram-negative and Gram-positive bacteria, although their envelope is regarded to be Gram-negative. Spirochetes of the genus *Borrelia* exhibit a complex life style, characterized by the ability to shuttle between hematophagous arthropods and various vertebrates, which exposes them to a variety of niches that are different in nutritional composition as well as immunological pressure. Survival, transmission and ultimately pathogenesis during infection obviously require a large degree of adaptive biological capacity. Thus, the interactions between the host and *Borrelia* pathogens need to be optimized for interaction with different environments such as the tick midgut, and various mammalian tissues. The different surface-exposed proteins play an important role in this process by providing ligands for receptor-mediated adhesion, mechanisms of host immune response avoidance, as well as pathways for the acquisition of nutrients.

Borreliae are considered to be Gram-negative bacteria because they possess two membranes and a periplasmic peptidoglycan layer, which in *Borrelia* is anchored to the inner membrane [1]. In spite of this, if *Borrelia* are compared to typical Gram-negative bacteria such as *Escherichia coli*, their cell envelope differs in many aspects (Fig. 1). While flagella in typical Gram-negative bacteria are placed on the surface of the outer membrane, the flagella in *Borreliae* are found in the periplasmic space between inner and outer membranes. This peculiar characteristic is shared among the spirochetes. Another large difference between the common Gram-negative eubacteria and *Borreliae* spirochetes is the absence of lipopolysaccharides [2, 3]. Instead, the outer membrane in *Borreliae* is very rich in lipoproteins, which represent the primary interface between the bacterium and the host [4]. The borrelial outer membranes are considerably more fluid than those of other Gram negative bacteria. They also possess a lower density of membrane spanning proteins [5, 6]. Porins, the focus of this review, are also found in the outer membrane of spirochetes with remarkably unique characteristics.

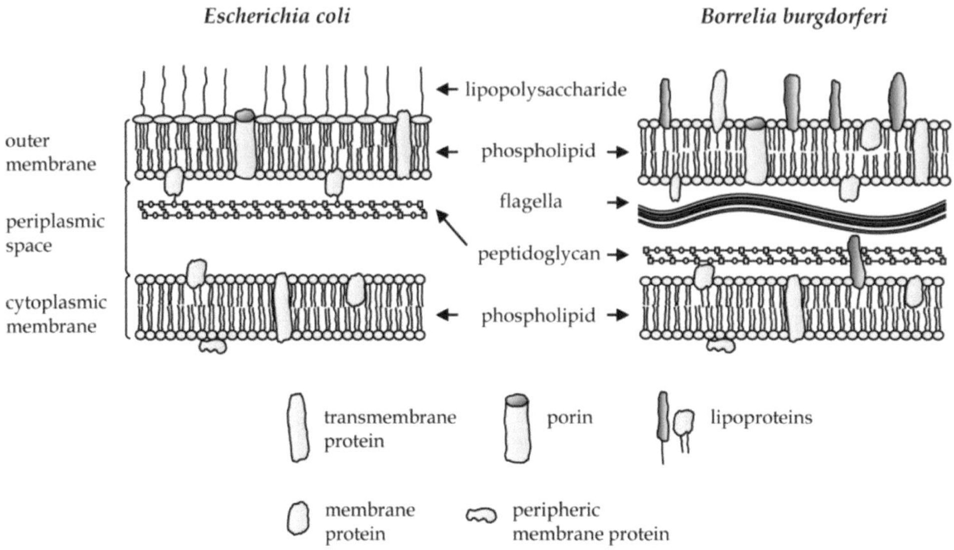

Fig. 1. Comparison of the cell envelope of a typical Gram negative bacterium such as *Escherichia coli* and *Borrelia burgdorferi*. While *E. coli* has a high content of lipopolysaccharides in its outer membrane, *B. burgdorferi* has a high amount of lipoproteins. Periplasmic flagella and a lower amount of external membrane spanning proteins are also typical *Borrelia* features.

1.1.1 Lipoproteins in the outer membrane of *Borrelia*

The protein content of the borrelial outer membrane is represented by a huge quantity of lipoproteins. As an indication of their importance in *Borrelia*, lipoproteins are the most abundant proteins in these species [7]. These proteins are located on the surface of the bacterial cell and anchored in the outer leaflet of the outer membrane. Borrelial lipoproteins play a major role in the activation of the innate immune response of the host as well as in the adaptive responses and pathogenicity of *Borrelia* spirochetes. Thus, this class of proteins is responsible for the activation of host inflammatory response as tissue inflammation which is a unifying feature during the manifestation of Lyme disease. Lipoproteins dominate pathogenicity mechanisms exploited by *B. burgdorferi*, including antigenic variation [8, 9], evasion of complement killing [10-12] and adhesion mechanisms [13].

The most abundant and best described outer membrane lipoproteins in the Lyme disease species *B. burgdorferi* are the so-called outer surface proteins (Osps). The most prominent lipoprotein species is OspA. OspA tertiary structure contains a single-layer β-sheet connecting the N- and C-terminal globular domains [14]. OspA acts as an adhesin in the tick environment [15] and it could have a protective function for P66 against proteases [16]. OspC, another well-studied *B. burgdorferi* lipoprotein, is homologous to variable small proteins (Vsps) of relapsing fever *Borrelia* [17]. The tertiary structure of OspC is also known and differs completely from OspA/B. It basically consists of five parallel α-helices and two short β-strands [18, 19]. This lipoprotein seems to be required to infect mice [20]. Interestingly, the OspA/B and OspC expression is reciprocally regulated and undergoes a switch during spirochete transition from the tick vector to the mammalian host. Thus, the

OspA expression is up-regulated in unfed ticks while OspC is expressed in large amounts in feeding ticks and in the mammalian host [21].

Beside the Osps, there is a wide variety of lipoproteins with different functionalities present in *B. burgdorferi*, such as the multicopy lipoproteins Mlps [22], Lp6.6, a small lipoprotein of 6.6 kDa [23], the decorin-binding proteins DbpA/B [24], the glycosaminoglycan-binding protein Bgp [25], P35 comprising two lipoproteins [26], the Vmp-like-sequence Vls [27], the Bmp family [28], P22 [29], the OspE/F related proteins Erps [30], the Elps containing OspE/F-like leader peptides [30] and the complement regulator acquiring surface proteins CRASPs [10].

In contrast to Lyme disease species, the most abundant proteins in the relapsing fever species' outer membranes are the variable major proteins Vmp. These lipoproteins are expressed with different surface epitopes through antigenic variation [31-33]. The lipoproteins of relapsing fever agents are subdivided into two families: the variable large proteins (Vlps) and the variable small proteins (Vsps) [7, 34, 35]. Interestingly, the expression of the single Vsp species is correlated to the pattern and the state of the disease. Vsps undergo antigenic variation and at least three mechanisms are known for surface alteration of relapsing fever lipoproteins [36, 37].

1.2 Porins in gram-negative bacteria

Porins are a group of proteins located in the outer membrane of Gram negative bacteria that facilitate the transfer of substances in both directions between the surrounding environment and the periplasmic space. Porins are also found in mycobacteria, chloroplasts and mitochondria [38, 39].

Porins form water-filled channels that allow a passive transport of molecules down their concentration gradients [40, 41]. This transport through the outer membrane does not require energy in contrast to the uphill substrate translocation via transporters in the inner membrane.

Most of the porins described to date form β barrels composed of antiparallel β-sheets. Frequently, they are associated in oligomers that confer a higher stability to the whole complex (Fig. 2). In the outer membrane of Gram negative bacteria, channel-tunnel proteins like TolC in *Escherichia* and BesC in *Borrelia* are also found. They form pores in the outer membrane and are part of bigger protein complexes involved in drug-resistance known as efflux pumps (Fig.2).

Porins can be classified in two groups depending on whether they are selective for a class of molecules or not [42]:

General diffusion porins allow the transport of small molecules, ions and water through a membrane. The permeability of general diffusion pores for substrates is dependent only on their size and charge. Examples for this kind of porins are OmpF and OmpC of *E. coli* [40].

Substrate-specific porins represent pores or channels that are specialized for the transport of certain molecules. These molecules bind to the channel interior and are guided to the periplasm. Tsx is an example of a substrate specific porin in *E. coli* that is specialized in the nucleoside transport from the surrounding media to the periplasmic space (Fig. 2) [43, 44]. Other examples include porins with specificity for carbohydrates [45], phosphate [46] and antibiotics [47].

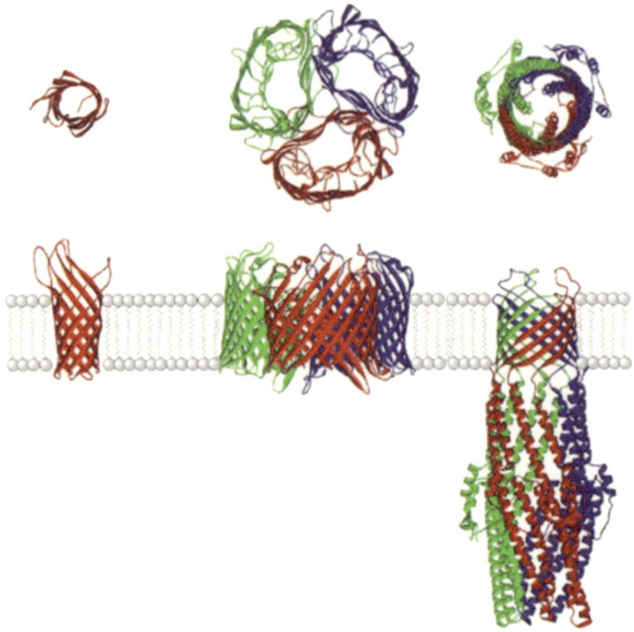

Fig. 2. Bacterial outer-membrane pore-forming proteins. Diffusion channels have usually a β-barrel tertiary structure with longer loops to the outside and short turns towards the periplasmic space. In *E. coli*, Tsx is a substrate specific porin for nucleosides while OmpC is a general diffusion porin. Usually porins form trimers like OmpC although other associations are also possible like in the case of Tsx. TolC is a channel-tunnel that together with an inner membrane transport system and adaptor proteins forms an efflux pump for export of drugs and other substances. These channel-tunnels are also formed by trimers but they only form a single pore.

2. Porins in the genus *Borrelia*

Borrelia species possess a small genome composed of a small linear chromosome complemented with a set of up to 21 linear and circular plasmids [48]. Many of their genes are related to bacterial virulence and the adaptation of bacteria to the different hosts and vectors. The absence of genes in *Borrelia* involved in the biosynthesis of amino acids, fatty acids or nucleotides is very remarkable. This metabolic deficiency makes *Borrelia* species strictly dependent on substances provided by their host. Therefore, the role of the *Borrelia* porins in the acquisition of nutrients is of extreme importance.

Up to now, five porins and a channel-tunnel as part of a multi-drug efflux system have been described in the outer membrane of different *Borreliae*. P66, P13, BBA01 (a P13 paralogue) and BBA74 have been described in *Borrelia burgdorferi*. Oms38 has been described in relapsing fever species, and possess a homologue in *Borrelia burgdorferi* designated DipA. Another outer membrane pore-forming protein is BesC. BesC is a channel-tunnel which is part of a bigger complex spanning the whole cell envelope which is involved in secretion of toxic compounds for *Borrelia*, like for example antibiotics.

2.1 P66: A porin with an unusual high single channel conductance

P66 exhibits a dual function. P66 is a well-studied pore-forming outer membrane protein present in Lyme disease and relapsing fever *Borreliae* [49-55]. Interestingly, P66 exhibits dual functions. It was shown to act as an adhesin which can bind to β(1)- and β(3)-chain integrins [51-53]. And strikingly, it acts as a porin in the outer membrane with the capability of forming pores with an extremely high single-channel conductance. This could be demonstrated by studies in planar lipid membranes [50, 54, 55]. In addition, P66 is also of special interest because of the presence of surface-exposed loops [49, 56] exhibiting a certain immunogenic potential [57], a property of interest in the search of vaccine candidates against European LD *Borreliae*.

P66 is present in both Lyme disease and relapsing fever agents. Comparison of the deduced P66 amino acid sequences from published genomes of the Lyme disease species *B. burgdorferi* B31, *B. afzelii* pKo, *B. garinii* PBi and the relapsing fever species *B. duttonii* Ly, *B. recurrentis* A1 and *B. hermsii* HS1 revealed 41% inter-species identity with partially highly conserved domains. The three LD species' P66 share the high sequence identity of 90%. P66 has according to its name a molecular weight of 66 kDa as can be seen after SDS-PAGE of purified P66.

P66 exhibits an unusually high single channel conductance. The pore-forming properties of P66 channels from the LD species *B. burgdorferi*, *B. afzelii* and *B. garinii* have been studied in detail by different groups [50, 54, 55]. P66 is able to form pores in planar lipid bilayers with the enormously high single-channel conductance of 11 nS in 1 M KCl [55]. Thereby, the conductance for P66 of the LD species *B. burgdorferi*, *B. afzelii*, *B. garinii* in 1 M KCl were all similarly high, in a range between 9 and 11 nS [55]. Measurements in different KCl concentrations from 0.1 to 3 M revealed that the single channel conductance was approximately a linear function of the electrolyte concentration which indicates a lack of binding sites for ions.

The P66 channels are nonselective for small anions and cations [50, 55]. This was demonstrated by single-channel experiments with salts containing cations and anions of different size such as LiCl and KCH_3COO and by the analysis of the membrane potential using the Goldman-Hodgin-Katz equation [58]. P66 channels are permeable for both anions and cations, because the calculated values of the permeability ratio of cations over anions (P_c/P_a) in KCl were in the range between 0.8 and 1.0 for all measured P66 homologues [55]. Values close to one indicate equal pore permeability for anions and cations.

P66 channels exhibit voltage-dependent closure. This was demonstrated in multi-channel experiments. *B. burgdorferi* P66 started to show voltage-dependent closure at potentials as high as + 70 and -60 mV reaching a maximal conductance decrease of approximately 20%. P66 homologues of different LD species all showed similar voltage-dependent behavior with slight species-specific differences of the potential for the start of conductance decrease. For example, for P66 of *B. afzelii* and *B. garinii*, the voltage-dependent closure started at potentials as high as +/- 40 mV and the conductance decreased by approximately 30% at applied potentials of +/-80 mV and higher [55].

The pore diameter of P66 is small related to the huge single-channel conductance. The above mentioned outstanding high single-channel conductance of 11 nS (in 1 M KCl) is atypical and rare for Gram-negative bacterial porins. However, certain spirochetal porins exhibit also an extremely high single-channel conductance, such as the one of the major outer membrane protein of *Spirochaeta aurantia*, which forms pores with a conductance of 7.7 nS in 1 M KCl [59] and the one of the major surface protein of *Treponema denticola*, Msp, a 53 kDa species (forming 1.8 nS pores in 0.1 M KCl) [60]. So far, beside selectivity and estimated pore diameters, very little is understood about the pore size and the structure of these outer membrane channels. In terms of P66, the channel diameter was calculated to be about 2.6 nm based on the assumption that the conductance of the channel is equal to the conductivity of a simple cylinder of aqueous salt solution [50]. This would be a rather large diameter compared to other pore-forming outer membrane proteins [61]. Anyway, the calculated value of the P66 diameter appears to be rather preliminary and theoretical.

Hence, the question arises what is the apparent channel diameter of P66 and its molecular organization in the outer membrane of *Borrelia* species. This question was answered by conductance measurements of the P66 channel reconstituted in planar lipid membranes in the presence of non-charged molecules, so-called nonelectrolytes (NEs), and the conductance was studied as a function of the size of the spherical NEs (Thein et al. unpublished). When the NEs can enter the P66 channel they will reduce its conductance as has been shown previously [62]. This means that the molecular mass cut-off for NEs and their hydrodynamic radii could provide a measure of the pore diameter [62].

Single-channel measurements with P66 in the presence of NEs revealed that NEs with a hydrodynamic radius (r) $\leq$ 0.8 nm enter the pore whereas NEs with r $\geq$ 0.94 nm are not permeable and cannot enter the P66 channel (Thein et al. unpublished). Evaluation of these data obtained with a method described by Krasilnikov et al. 1998 [63] indicated that the precise value of the effective P66 radius is about 0.94 $\pm$ 0.1 nm (Thein et al. unpublished). This means that P66 has an effective pore diameter of less than 1.9 nm, a value which is significantly smaller than the prediction of 2.6 nm [50]. Thus, P66 has an apparent channel diameter close to the one of several other Gram-negative bacterial porins and other membrane channels [63-65], that were characterized by the use of NEs. But one has to consider that the P66 single-channel conductance is up to 60-fold higher than the single-channel conductance of those channels with a comparable channel diameter (Thein et al. unpublished).

The molecular organization of P66 seems to be peculiar. This discrepancy between single-channel conductance and effective diameter suggests that the channel-forming domain of P66 is based on an outstanding molecular organization. And indeed, when P66 is subjected to a Blue Native PAGE, a 440 kDa protein band can be observed. This means that P66 can indeed form a hexamer or a heptamer in its membrane-active configuration because seven 66 kDa monomers could form an oligomer with a calculated molecular mass of approximately 460 kDa. This finding is supported by conductance measurements of one single P66 unit. After reconstitution of one single 11 nS unit, the defined single-channel conductance of P66, in the membrane, the ionic current through the channel can be substantially blocked by the addition of 90 mM PEG 400. And strikingly, this blockage occurs stepwise in seven closing substates (Fig. 3) (Thein et al. unpublished). The conductance of all those substates is fairly homogenous and is on average about 1.5 nS. The substate conductance of 1.5 nS confirms the Blue Native PAGE result, because seven 1.5 nS substates yield a conductance in the range of 11 nS. This means that the individual P66 molecules are forming a high molecular mass protein complex: The individual channels in the oligomer act like molecular sieves with an exclusion size of approximately 1.9 nm. These findings have not been observed for typical porins of Gram-negative bacteria (Thein et al. unpublished).

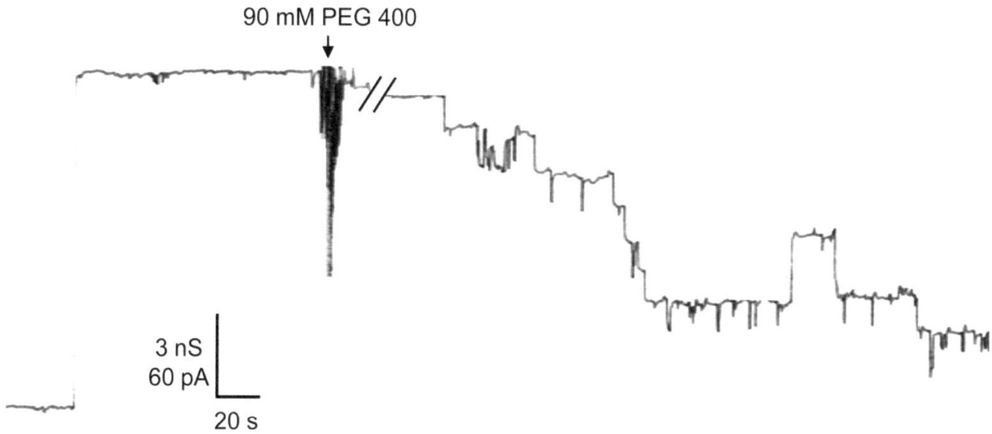

Fig. 3. Blockage steps of a single P66 channel after addition of PEG 400. A single P66 channel was reconstituted in a diphytanoyl phosphatidylcholine artificial membrane embedded in a 1M KCl salt solution. Some time after addition of PEG 400 the channel was blocked in several steps, each one corresponding probably to an independent channel subunit.

2.2 P13: An atypical α-helical porin

P13 is a surface-exposed epitope. In 1995 Sadziene et al. [66] described an accessible protein in a *B. burgdorferi* strain called *B. burgdorferi* B313 lacking several lipoproteins. In this study the inactivation of four lipoproteins, OspA, OspB, OspC and OspD, in *Borrelia burgdorferi* B31 and its posterior inoculation in a rodent triggered an immune response against a surface exposed 13 kDa protein [66]. This antibody had no influx in the growth of a native strain highlighting a possible P13 protective function of these mutated lipoproteins. To study the effect of this antibody on cell growth, the B313 mutant was compared with another mutant, B311, where only two lipoproteins, OspC and OspD, were mutated. The MIC of this antibody for the B311 stain was more than 600-fold higher than for the B313, revealing a possible P13 protective function of OspA and/or OspB against the immune system [66]. This protective function of some lipoproteins for transmembrane proteins has also been described for other *Borrelia* proteins [16].

Other experiments treating *Borrelia* cells with proteinase K and trypsin confirmed the exposure of P13 to the surrounding media [67]. Further immunofluorescence assay and immunogold-labeling confirmed again the homogeneous distribution of P13 in the outer membrane of *Borrelia burgdorferi* [67]. The surface exposure of P13 and the lack of any other known homologue in other living organisms makes this protein a perfect candidate to be used in new diagnosis and therapeutic strategies [67].

P13 permeabilized lipid membranes similarly as bacterial porins. Purification to homogeneity followed by black lipid bilayer experiments revealed a pore forming activity for P13. Single channel insertions in artificial membranes displayed a conductance of 3.5 nS in 1 M KCl [68]. Further analysis of the P13 pore forming activity revealed that the channel was slightly cation selective and voltage independent [68]. No specific substrate has been found for P13 although titration experiments had been carried out with different sugars, amino acids and other relevant substrates (Bárcena-Uribarri et al. unpublished data). For these reasons P13 is considered to be a general diffusion porin with a quite stable structure.

P13 is posttranslationally processed and modified on its N- and C-termini. Mass spectrometry analysis of mature P13 located in the outer membrane revealed a molecular mass of 13,968 ±1 Da. This fact was consistent with the molecular mass estimations by SDS-Page and Tricine-SDS-Page. N-terminal and C-terminal sequencing of the protein revealed a blocked N-terminus and a processed C-terminus that lacked the last 28 amino acids [67, 69]. A pyroglutamic acid modification was later proven to be present at the N- terminus [69]. Computer predictions for a Signal Peptidase I cleavage site after amino acid 19 in the N-terminus were consistent with the predicted molecular mass for mature P13.

P13 is processed at the C-terminal end in the periplasmic space. Another remarkable peculiarity of P13 is the C-terminal peptide that is cleaved in the periplasmic space by CtpA [70]. This kind of caboxyl-terminal proteases have also been identified in other bacteria [71] including an homologue in *E. coli* [72] and in chloroplasts of algae and higher plants [73, 74]. In *Borrelia burgdorferi*, the CtpA is the responsible for the cleavage of 28 amino acids in the C-terminal end of P13. The CtpA protease has also an influence on the expression of several other proteins, such as BB0323 and Oms28. CtpA has a signal sequence for the transport to the periplasmic space and therefore the processing of the C-terminus of P13 is believed to happen in the periplasmic space [70].

The aim of the C-terminal processing and a possible function of the C-terminal peptide of P13 is unknown. However, a mutant of the CtpA protease showed that this processing is not required to localize P13 in the outer membrane of *Borrelia* [70]. Whether the P13 has to be processed to form a protein complex or if the P13 peptide has its own function has not been clarified yet.

No lipidation or glycosylation was found to occur in P13. A potential leader peptidase II cleavage-lipid modification was found in the P13 sequence. However, experiments with radio-labeled fatty acids or immunoblots for glycoprotein detection showed no apparent modification of P13 by fatty acids or carbohydrates [67]

P13 is an α-helical transmembrane protein. Initial experiments predicted three α-helical transmembrane domains for P13 based on computer modeling. When the model was compared to other strain sequences it could be observed that the hypothetical transmembrane domains were highly conserved while the exposed loops regions were more variable [67]. This fact is in agreement with a surface exposure of the loops that undergo a higher immune pressure. Later on, this hypothesis was tested with an experimental approach where three fragments of mature P13 were designed and produced recombinant. Based on the computer model two were transmembrane domains and one corresponded to the external loop. Only the segment though to be the external loop was recognized by an antibody that strictly recognizes the natural epitope of the P13 protein confirming this hypothesis (Fig. 4) [66, 75].

The P13 oligomeric structure does not follow the typical model of a bacterial porin. Most of the 3D-structures of porins show β-barrel cylinders often organized as trimers [76]. Each monomer forms an individual channel that acquires a higher stability in association with two other identical units. In the case of P13 its small size makes the formation of a channel by itself improbable and an oligomeric quaternary structure is required to form a channel in

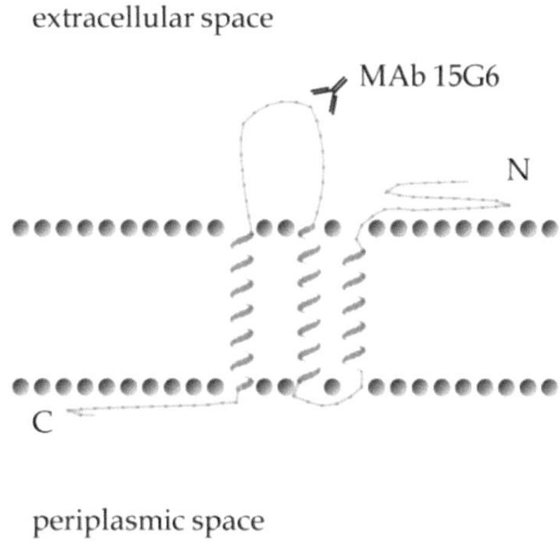

Fig. 4. P13 predicted secondary structure. Computer modeling and some experimental approaches disclose three α-helical transmembrane domains. An external loop is placed to the outside and it is the antigenic determinant for the Mab 15G6 antibody, which recognizes the surface-exposed region of P13 in "*in vivo*" immunolabeling.

the outer membrane of *Borrelia*. Some indications of P13 oligomerization have been previously described but the exact number of monomers involved in this protein complex remains still unclear [68]. The P13 α-helical secondary structure is also not typical for bacterial porins. Only a few examples of α-helical porins have been described, all of them in Gram-positive bacteria and none of them with monomers spanning the membrane three times as supposed for P13 (Fig. 4) [77, 78]. These features make P13 to a possible new kind of pore forming protein not described before for any other bacteria.

The P13 C-terminal peptide has high pore-forming activity in artificial membranes. The P13 C-terminal peptide has been tested with the black lipid bilayer assay to check its pore-forming capacity. This small 28 amino acid peptide displayed a pore forming capacity with pores that vary in conductance from the pS range to bigger than 20 nS (Bárcena-Uribarri et al., unpublished results). A potential toxicity of this C-terminus for mammalian cells has still to be tested.

2.2.1 The paralogue family 48: The BBA01 protein

Eight P13 paralogues have been found within the genome of *Borrelia burgdorferi*, constituting the paralogue family [48]. P13 is a protein encoded in the main chromosome of *Borrelia.* All the paralogues are encoded in linear plasmids, some of them carrying two copies. Two of these paralogues are pseudogenes and do not produce functional proteins. A third paralogue displays an authentic frameshift producing a different protein and the other five produce conserved hypothetical proteins. BBA01 is from all of them the closest paralogue to P13 with a 54.1 % similarity on the amino acid level [79].

BBA01 displays porin activity and it is potentially interchangeable with P13. The recombinant expression and purification of BBA01 in *E. coli* revealed a porin activity similar to the one described for P13 [79]. An up-regulation of BBA01 in a P13 mutant raised the hypothesis of a possible function compensation of P13 [79].

2.3 BBA74: Oms28 a controversial porin

BBA74, also known as Oms28, was first described as a porin in the outer membrane of *Borrelia burgdorferi*. In 1995 Skare et al. described two pore-forming activities in the outer membrane vesicles coming from *Borrelia burgdorferi* [80]. The conductance of these two porins was 0.6 and 12.6 nS. A posterior study where the different proteins were isolated in different fractions by FPLC and SDS-Page elution attributed the 0.6 nS activity to a 28 kDa protein (Fig. 5) [81]. This protein was designated as outer membrane-spanning protein of 28 kDa, Oms28.

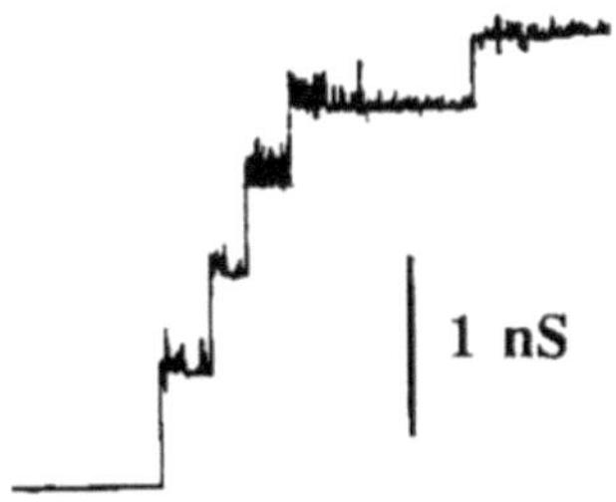

Fig. 5. Pore forming activity of 0.6 nS coming from outer membrane vesicles preparations of *Borrelia burgdorferi*. After isolation of outer membrane vesicles and further purification a clear 0.6 nS activity could be observed. This pore forming activity was attributed to BBA74. Taken from ref. [81] by permission.

The pore forming activity of Oms28 can be regained after separation in SDS-PAGE showing some resistant of this protein to the detergent SDS. Interestingly, certain oligomeric forms were observed after reducing the concentration of the detergent, removal of β-mercaptoethanol from the sample buffer and avoiding boiling prior electrophoresis [81].

Recombinant expression of BBA74 showed a similar pore-forming activity to the native protein. Recombinant production of BBA074 in *E. coli* and its posterior separation by SDS-PAGE and elution from the gel displayed a 1.1 nS pore forming activity. Native BBA074 has a 0.6 nS pore-forming activity. Possible explanations for the difference in conductance of the recombinant protein are an alteration in the tertiary structure folding or the preferential insertion as dimers [81].

BBA74 is transported to the periplasm. Computer analysis of the BBA74 protein sequence revealed a 24 amino acid signal sequence with a peptidase I cleavage site [81]. As described for outer membrane proteins BBA74 has a signal sequence to be transported from the cytoplasm to the periplasm. The initial protein of 28 kDa yields a mature protein of 25.3 kDa after the transport through the inner membrane and the cleavage of the signal sequence [81].

The association of BBA74 with the outer membrane resulted in some discrepancies in different studies. Skare et al. [81] showed the BBA74 association with the outer membrane by treating *Borrelia* cells with harsh salt solutions. BBA74 was retained in the membrane pellet as expected for integral membrane proteins [81]. Controversially, in cells subjected to Triton X-114 phase partitioning BBA74 partitioned exclusively into the aqueous phase whereas typical transmembrane proteins stay in the detergent phase [81, 82]. These results have to be considered with some caution because Pinne and Haake [83] demonstrated in a independent study that Triton X-114 can be problematic for the localization of outer membrane spanning proteins in spirochetes and these investigations need to be complemented with other methods to address this question accurately [83].

BBA74 lacks typical porin features. To complement the information about the possible localization of BBA74 additional experiments were performed. Its secondary structure was study by CD spectroscopy revealing a vast majority of α-helical folding [82]. The surface exposure of BBA74 was investigated by proteinase K digestion and immunofluorescence microscopy. No digestion of BBA74 or fluorescence could be observed in wild type strains of *B. burgdorferi* indicating that this protein has no accessible surface-exposed regions [82]. Usually bacterial porins partition in the detergent fraction when treated with Triton X-114, they have a β-barrel tertiary structure and they have some accessible surface exposed loops. Because BBA74 lacks this properties it has been hypothesized that it could be a protein only associated to the inner leaflet of the outer membrane.

Extracellular secretion of BBA74 has been described. Radiolabeled amino acids were used to study the secretion of proteins in *B. burgdorferi*. Free protein medium was supplemented with radiolabeled methionine and cysteine. After some growing time the cells and the medium were separated by centrifugation. In the medium some proteins were found, among them BBA74 (Oms28) and Bgp [84]. This fact supports the hypothesis of a possible BBA74 extracellular secretion.

However, it is known that *Borrelia* releases outer membrane vesicles and blebs containing BBA74, OspA and OspB under stressful conditions. To rule out the possibility of this being the cause for the detection of BBA74 in the media, immunoblots against these three proteins were carried out. While BBA74 was found in the cells and in the free-protein medium, OspA-B were only found in the cell pellet [84].

BBA74 was mainly secreted during the mid- to late-logarithmic phase. In the same study dealing with a possible secretion of BBA74 its secretion pattern was examined. Recollection of samples during the growing process revealed that BBA74 expression was at its highest level during the logarithmic phase while during the stationary-phase the amount of BBA74 was considerably smaller [84].

The *bba74* gene is transcribed exclusively during larval and nymphal blood meals. The sigma factor 70 is responsible for its transcription while RpoS independent and dependent mechanisms stops the transcription in response to arthropod and mammalian host-specific signals [85].

BBA74 is not expressed during murine infection and the loss of the gene does not seem to affect the infectivity or the transit between the tick and the mouse [85].

2.4 DipA / Oms38: A specific porin for dicarboxylates

In contrast to the general diffusion porin P66 with its huge single-channel conductance, DipA is a substrate-specific porin and exhibits a very small single-channel conductance. DipA is responsible for the rapid influx of compounds belonging to the dicarboxylates (Thein et al. unpublished).

DipA was first identified in knock-out mutants of *B. burgdorferi*, *B. burgdorferi* Δp66 and *B. burgdorferi* Δp13/Δp66 [54]. During black lipid bilayer experiments with isolated outer membranes of those mutants, high channel-forming activities in the conductance range between 10 and 100 pS were detected, which could not be related to one of the previously described OM pores P13, Oms28, P66 and BesC. This finding indicated the presence of a porin with a small single-channel conductance in the outer membrane. Interestingly, after subjecting the outer membrane fraction of *B. burgdorferi* to hydroxyapatite chromatography, a pore-forming protein could be purified with an apparent molecular mass of 36 kDa (Thein et al. unpublished).

Mass-spectrometric analysis of the protein revealed its sequence and confirmed it to be a homologue of the Oms38 porin of relapsing fever *Borreliae* [86]. The deduced amino acid sequence contains an N-terminal cleavage site, which is typical for proteins localized in the outer membrane. The localization in the outer membrane was confirmed by electron-micrographs of immunogold-labeled *B. burgdorferi* cells decorated with antibodies against the identified 36 kDa protein. Computational analysis of the deduced amino acid sequence predicted putative ß-strands, which suggested that the secondary structure of DipA may contain many ß-sheets similar as is known for the ß-barrel cylinders of well-studied bacterial porins [87, 88]. All these findings indicated the identification of another porin in *B. burgdorferi*, and the protein was consequently named DipA, which stands for "dicarboxylate-specific porin A", due to its function as a dicarboxylate-specific porin (see below) (Thein et al. unpublished).

DipA was extensively characterized in the black lipid bilayer assay (Thein et al. unpublished): it forms pores in the artificial membrane which exhibit a small single-channel conductance of 50 pS in 1 M KCl. DipA pores were also investigated for voltage-dependent behavior. In the range from -120 V to +120 V the voltage does not show any influence on the conductance demonstrating that DipA is not voltage-dependent up to these potentials (Thein et al. unpublished).

DipA is a porin selective for anions. This was shown by multi-channel experiments under zero-current potential conditions. The permeability ratios of cations over anions through DipA were calculated from the zero-current potentials using the Goldman-Hodgkin-Katz equation [58]. They revealed together with the zero-current membrane potential that DipA is preferentially anion selective, because the ratios of the permeability coefficients P_{cation}/P_{anion} were 0.57 (in KCl), 0.47 (in LiCl). The P_{cation}/P_{anion} in KCH_3COO was 1.65, which means that also cations have certain permeability through the DipA pore (Thein et al. unpublished).

Strikingly, the DipA single-channel conductance of 50 pS is much smaller than the one of typical general diffusion pores [76]. This small single-channel conductance and the fact that growth of *Borrelia* is highly dependent on the uptake of nutrients [89, 90] suggests that DipA is a channel specific for essential nutrients and contains a binding site for them in a similar way as the carbohydrate-specific *E. coli* channel LamB [91, 92]. This hypothesis was tested by titration experiments using different classes of substrates as described previously for titration of LamB with carbohydrates [45, 92]. Interestingly, many classes of substrates that are necessary for bacterial growth including carbohydrates, such as glucose, fructose, sucrose, maltose and lactose, nucleosides, such as adenosine, and other anionic molecules, like acetate, carbonate, phosphate and adenosine triphosphate, do not show any interaction with DipA. Interestingly, DipA can be partly blocked by dicarboxylates (Thein et al. unpublished).

DipA-mediated channel-conductance can be partly blocked by addition of dicarboxylates. After DipA channel reconstitution into lipid bilayer membranes and having an approximately stationary membrane conductance, concentrated solutions of different dicarboxylates were added to the aqueous phase at both sides of the membrane. As a consequence, the DipA-mediated membrane conductance was dose-dependently blocked. For example, the the DipA conductance decreases by 23% after addition of malate, 29% after addition of 2-oxoglutarate and 25% in after addition of phthalate at substrate concentrations of 27 mM, 9 mM and 4 mM, respectively (Fig. 6). Strikingly, DipA can be blocked by a variety of dicarboxylates and other related organic anions with high biological relevance. The tested compounds include oxaloacetate, succinate, malate, fumarate, maleate, 2-oxoglutarate, phthalate, citrate, aspartate, glutamate, and pyruvate. All anions listed previously block the ion current through DipA with a maximum block of channel conductance ranging from 20% for pyruvate to 31% for oxaloacetate (Thein et al. unpublished).

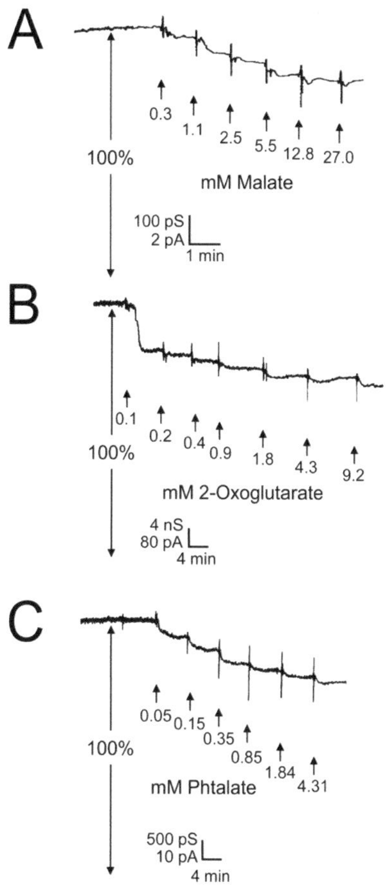

Fig. 6. Titrations of DipA-mediated conductance with different dicarboxylates. Membranes saturated with DipA were titrated with increasing concentrations of A) Malate, B) 2-Oxoglutarate, C) Phtalate. (Thein et al., unpublished). The binding of these molecules to the channel interior slows the translocation of KCl because of partial blocking of ion flux through the channel.

From these titration experiments, the binding affinities of the tested dicarboxylates to DipA were analyzed in a similar way as used for the characterization of carbohydrate-binding channels of Gram-negative bacteria [45, 92]. Binding of dicarboxylates to DipA yield high stability constants for oxaloacetate (K = 19,900 ± 5,100 l/mol), succinate (K = 6,100 ± 2,200 l/mol), malate (K = 1,300 ± 520 l/mol), maleate (K = 28,300 ± 950l/mol) and 2-oxoglutarate (K = 3,500 ± 140 l/mol). This means that binding of the tested compounds to the DipA channel show a significant specificity. The detailed study of the DipA specificity revealed that the stability constants depended strongly on the specific structure of the organic anion showing a maximum for C4-dicarboxylates oxaloacetate and maleate. The binding specificities to certain substrates are distinctly depending on the number of carboxylic acid groups and on side groups of the anions like oxo-, hydroxyl- or amino- groups (Thein et al. unpublished).

In analogy to other bacterial specific porins, it is likely that the DipA binding site with its high affinity for dicarboxylic anions increases the permeability of the channel for these metabolites as has been demonstrated previously: The presence of a binding site leads to an accelerated transport of carbohydrate through LamB and of phosphate transport through OprP, especially at very low substrate concentrations [40, 45]. Thus, the permeability of a substrate-specific porin can surpass that of a general diffusion pore by orders of magnitude in spite of its smaller cross-section [45].

Dicarboxylates, such as malate, succinate, oxaloacetate and 2-oxoglutarate, are major intermediates of the tricarboxylic acid cycle and are also used for synthesis of amino acids. For example, oxaloacetate and 2-oxoglutarate are important substrates for the biosynthesis of asparagine, aspartic acid and glutamic acid, respectively, which are essential proteinogenic amino acids. In addition, C4 dicarboxylates other than succinate cannot be metabolized due to the lack of a functional tricarboxylic acid cycle in anaerobic energy metabolism of most bacteria [93]. Taking these points into consideration, a potential dependence of the growth of *Borrelia* on this group of chemicals is likely. This hypothesis is additionally supported by the fact that the serum-supplemented mammalian tissue-culture medium for in vitro cultivation of *Borreliae* is supplemented by pyruvate and the tricarboxylic citrate. Amongst others, these compounds have been shown to specifically bind to DipA. Consequently DipA plays an important role in the uptake of dicarboxylates and related compounds across the outer membrane.

3. BesC: A channel-tunnel part of an efflux pump in the genus *Borrelia*

Many bacteria live in hostile environments where other organism or the infected hosts produce antimicrobial substances. To avoid possible toxicity of these compounds many bacteria have developed transport systems for export of harmful substances out of the cells called multi-drug resistance efflux systems [94, 95]. There are different types of these systems involved in the efflux of different substances like toxins, endogenous metabolic waste products or antibiotics. One of the most important multi-drug resistance efflux systems are the so called resistance-nodulation division (RND) transporters. This family of transporters is present in many living organisms but plays a crucial role in the export of toxic substances in Gram-negative bacteria.

The RND transporters in Gram-negative bacteria are composed of three components [95, 96]. An energy dependent transporter spanning the cytoplasmic membrane, a channel-tunnel crossing the outer membrane and the periplasmic space and a fusion protein located in the periplasmic space that connects both transporter and channel-tunnel. The best studied example of this kind of efflux pump is the multi-drug resistance pump AcrA-AcrB-TolC in *Escherichia coli*. In this case TolC is the protein situated in the outer membrane of *E. coli*, AcrB is thought to be a proton-driven translocase in the inner membrane and AcrA is the fusion protein connecting AcrB and TolC.

Only one study has been published about this type of systems in *Borrelia*. The *Borrelia burgdorferi* B31 genome sequencing allowed the identification of a TolC homologue called in *Borrelia* BesC (Fig. 7). The genes flanking this gene showed also high homology to AcrA and AcrB and they were called BesA and BesB respectively. The name of the genes Bes comes from *Borrelia* Efflux System. Analysis of the RNA coding for these genes showed that they were co-transcribed and transcriptional linked [97].

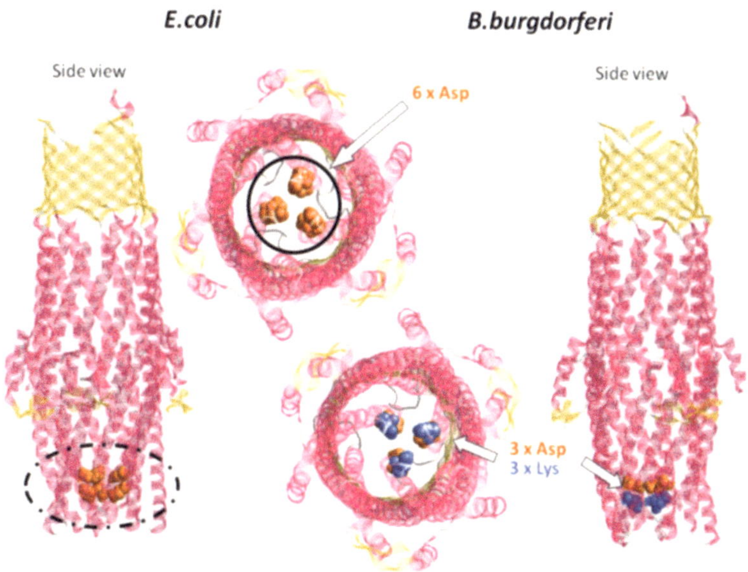

Fig. 7. Predicted 3D-structure of BesC based on TolC crystal structure [95]. Computer predictions for the structure of the TolC homologue BesC reveals a similar one as TolC. In contrast to TolC that has a positively charged periplasmic entrance, BesC has an entrance where positive and negative charges are compensated. Provided by Ignas Bunikis by courtesy.

BesC is essential for antibiotic resistance and necessary for mammal infection. A knock-out of the BesC gene resulted in a 2 to 64 fold decrease in the resistance to antibiotics compared to the wild type. Both the MIC (minimal inhibitory concentration) and MBC (minimal borreliacidal concentration) values were lowered by the lost of BesC [97]. Studies done in a mouse model showed that the BesC knock-out strain could not be recovered two weeks after mouse infection from heart, bladder, knee and ear biopsies. Whereas the knock-out strain was unable to survive in the mouse for that short period of time wild type and a complemented strain grew well in BSKII media after being collected from mice [97].

BesC forms pores in the outer membrane of *Borrelia*. Studies of BesC using the black lipid bilayer assay showed that BesC had an average single channel conductance of about 300 pS in 1M KCl at 20 mV transmembrane potential [97]. Channel-forming activity of pure BesC samples could be inactivated by their incubation with antibodies against BesC [97]. This provided further evidence that the channel-forming activity of the 300 pS channels were caused by BesC.

Biophysical studies of BesC suggested a slight anion selectivity and voltage independence. Zero-current membrane experiments were performed to study the ion selectivity of BesC. The increase of different salt concentrations in one of the membrane sides revealed no preference for translocation of anions or cations through the BesC channel [97]. Similarly, application of different positive and negative voltages up to 150 mV to a membrane saturated with BesC channels showed no reduction in the channel conductance revealing a very stable and voltage-independent channel [97].

The structure of BesC shows some differences to that of TolC [97]. Modeling of the BesC structure taking advantage of the known structure of TolC and TolC homologues revealed some variations especially at the N-terminal and C-terminal ends. A wider tunnel entrance in the BesC model could explain its 4-fold increased conductance in relation with TolC of *E. coli*. The missing ion selectivity of BesC could be explained by the substitution of one negatively charged aspartic acid residue by positively charged lysines at the periplasmic entrance of the three BesC monomers. The substitution of three negative charges at the entrance of the BesC trimer could counterbalance the residual three negative aspartates at the entrance, thus explaining the missing ion selectivity (Fig. 7).

All together there are five pore-forming proteins described in *Borrelia*. Four of them are porins and BesC is a channel-tunnel forming part of an efflux pump system. Pore forming proteins are usually characterized by different biophysical features such as its single channel conductance, ion selectivity, voltage dependence and possible specificities for substrates. The biophysical properties of P66, P13, BBA74, DipA and BesC are summarized in Table 1.

4. Conclusions

Spirochetes differ in many ways to other groups of bacteria. Similar to most bacteria, *Borrelia* obtain the nutrients from the surrounding media. The first step in the acquisition of essential substrates is their transport through the outer membrane. In all bacteria including *Borrelia* this transport is accomplished by protein channels located in the outer membrane named porins. However, the porins described so far in *Borrelia* seem to have special characteristics.

P66 is a special porin and remains an interesting research object, due to the fact that it shows a dual function as an adhesin and as a porin. Furthermore, it has an extremely high single-channel conductance and probably a peculiar molecular organization. Anyway, the exact molecular structure remains to be revealed by crystallization. Considering the high single-channel conductance of P66 and the organization as a molecular sieve with defined cut-off in the outer membrane of *Borrelia* cells, P66 seems to play a major role in the first import steps of general nutrients and other molecules.

P13 is probably one of the most intriguing proteins in *Borrelia*. Despite its small molecular weight and its secondary α-helical structure it forms channels in the outer membrane of *Borrelia*. The organization of P13 in protein complexes is required to form a channel given its small size. Apart from that, the presence of a periplasmic-cleaved C-terminal peptide which function is not completely understood is unique among porins. A very remarkable feature of P13 is the presence of up to eight paralogues in the genome of *Borrelia burgdorferi*. From those only BBA01 has been studied, showing similar pore forming characteristics as P13. The reason for the high number of copies for this gene is still not understood but it reinforces the idea of P13 being an essential outer membrane protein. The up regulation of BBA01 in a P13 knock-out to probably compensate its lack and the impossibility to obtain a P13-BBA01 double mutant reinforces this theory.

The function of BBA74 (Oms28) is controversial. It was described first as a porin with a single channel conductance of 0.6 nS. Its fractionation in the aqueous solution after treatment with Triton X-114 instead of in the detergent fraction where transmembrane proteins normally are found motivated later on an additional study. It concluded that BBA74 lacks the typical porin properties and it is just associated with the internal leaflet of the outer membrane. An independent study showed an extracellular secretion of BBA74 together with other proteins. This secretion seems to happen during the logarithmic growth phase and it is independent from the production of blebs or vesicles. Further studies are required to unify the knowledge of this protein and why the investigations created quite contradictory results.

Protein	M.W. [kDa]	Conductance [nS] in 1 M KCl	Selectivity	Voltage-dependence	Function
P66	66	11.0	not selective	yes	adhesin, porin
P13	13	3.5	for cations	no	porin
BBA074 (Oms28)	25	0.6	*n.d.*	no	porin-like properties?
DipA	36	0.05	for anions	no	dicarboxylate-specificity
BesC	48	0.3	not selective	*n.d.*	part of efflux- system

Table 1. Biophysical properties of the pore-forming proteins described in the outer membrane of *Borrelia burgdorferi*. M.W. means molecular weight of the processed protein; *n.d.* means not determined; conductance means average single-channel conductance measured in 1 M KCl.

DipA does not form general diffusion pores, but it is a specific porin. Its permeability properties are determined by charges in the channel that act like a filter. Thus, DipA is the first identified *Borrelia* porin exhibiting a substrate specificity and therefore has presumably a well-defined function in the biology of this spirochete. Its small conductance and its presence next to channels up to about two hundred times bigger such as P66 are very remarkable. This fact can only be explained by some kind of specificity of these channels for some indispensable substrates for *Borrelia*.

BesC is a well conserved homologue of the extensively studied TolC of *E. coli*. BesC forms part of a bigger complex similar as TolC that spans both membranes in *Borrelia*. This whole complex is involved in the export of toxic substances and antibiotics and plays presumably an important role for the infection in mammals.

The *Borrelia* porin research could have important consequences for the development of new strategies in diagnosis and vaccination to improve the treatment of infections by these bacteria. The ability of *Borrelia* to change their surface antigens and escape the immune system has made its correct diagnosis and treatment a really hard task. Surface-exposed essential proteins of the bacteria are the perfect candidates to be used as diagnosis/treatment targets. Porins could be used as ideal targets because they are important proteins for the biology of bacteria and can be fundamental in an infection procedure. The identification of the specific function, structure and expression profile of a porin is therefore relevant and a fascinating field to research on.

5. Acknowledgements

The authors would like to thank Ignas Bunikis for providing figure 7. This work was supported by the joint project between Stint (Sweden) and DAAD (Germany) to SB and RB, by the Deutsche Forschungsgemeinschaft to RB (project BE865/15) and the Swedish Medical Research Council to SB.

6. References

[1] Barbour, A.G. and S.F. Hayes, *Biology of Borrelia species.* Microbiol Rev, 1986. 50(4): p. 381-400.

[2] Takayama, K., R.J. Rothenberg, and A.G. Barbour, *Absence of lipopolysaccharide in the Lyme disease spirochete, Borrelia burgdorferi.* Infect Immun, 1987. 55(9): p. 2311-3.

[3] Belisle, J.T., et al., *Fatty acids of Treponema pallidum and Borrelia burgdorferi lipoproteins.* J Bacteriol, 1994. 176(8): p. 2151-7.

[4] Brandt, M.E., et al., *Immunogenic integral membrane proteins of Borrelia burgdorferi are lipoproteins.* Infect Immun, 1990. 58(4): p. 983-91.

[5] Walker, E.M., et al., *Analysis of outer membrane ultrastructure of pathogenic Treponema and Borrelia species by freeze-fracture electron microscopy.* J Bacteriol, 1991. 173(17): p. 5585-8.

[6] Radolf, J.D., et al., *Analysis of Borrelia burgdorferi membrane architecture by freeze-fracture electron microscopy.* J Bacteriol, 1994. 176(1): p. 21-31.

[7] Haake, D.A., *Spirochaetal lipoproteins and pathogenesis.* Microbiology, 2000. 146 (Pt 7): p. 1491-504.

[8] Zhang, J.R., et al., *Antigenic variation in Lyme disease borreliae by promiscuous recombination of VMP-like sequence cassettes.* Cell, 1997. 89(2): p. 275-85.

[9] Zhang, J.R. and S.J. Norris, *Genetic variation of the Borrelia burgdorferi gene vlsE involves cassette-specific, segmental gene conversion.* Infect Immun, 1998. 66(8): p. 3698-704.

[10] Kraiczy, P., et al., *Mechanism of complement resistance of pathogenic Borrelia burgdorferi isolates.* Int Immunopharmacol, 2001. 1(3): p. 393-401.

[11] Stevenson, B., et al., *Differential binding of host complement inhibitor factor H by Borrelia burgdorferi Erp surface proteins: a possible mechanism underlying the expansive host range of Lyme disease spirochetes.* Infect Immun, 2002. 70(2): p. 491-7.

[12] Alitalo, A., et al., *Complement inhibitor factor H binding to Lyme disease spirochetes is mediated by inducible expression of multiple plasmid-encoded outer surface protein E paralogs.* J Immunol, 2002. 169(7): p. 3847-53.

[13] Coburn, J., J.R. Fischer, and J.M. Leong, *Solving a sticky problem: new genetic approaches to host cell adhesion by the Lyme disease spirochete.* Mol Microbiol, 2005. 57(5): p. 1182-95.

[14] Li, H. and C.L. Lawson, *Crystallization and preliminary X-ray analysis of Borrelia burgdorferi outer surface protein A (OspA) complexed with a murine monoclonal antibody Fab fragment.* J Struct Biol, 1995. 115(3): p. 335-7.

[15] Pal, U., et al., *Attachment of Borrelia burgdorferi within Ixodes scapularis mediated by outer surface protein A.* J Clin Invest, 2000. 106(4): p. 561-9.

[16] Bunikis, J. and A.G. Barbour, *Access of antibody or trypsin to an integral outer membrane protein (P66) of Borrelia burgdorferi is hindered by Osp lipoproteins.* Infect Immun, 1999. 67(6): p. 2874-83.

[17] Carter, C.J., et al., *A family of surface-exposed proteins of 20 kilodaltons in the genus Borrelia.* Infect Immun, 1994. 62(7): p. 2792-9.
[18] Eicken, C., et al., *Crystal structure of Lyme disease antigen outer surface protein C from Borrelia burgdorferi.* J Biol Chem, 2001. 276(13): p. 10010-5.
[19] Kumaran, D., et al., *Crystal structure of outer surface protein C (OspC) from the Lyme disease spirochete, Borrelia burgdorferi.* EMBO J, 2001. 20(5): p. 971-8.
[20] Grimm, D., et al., *Outer-surface protein C of the Lyme disease spirochete: a protein induced in ticks for infection of mammals.* Proc Natl Acad Sci U S A, 2004. 101(9): p. 3142-7.
[21] de Silva, A.M., et al., *Borrelia burgdorferi OspA is an arthropod-specific transmission-blocking Lyme disease vaccine.* J Exp Med, 1996. 183(1): p. 271-5.
[22] Caimano, M.J., et al., *Molecular and evolutionary characterization of the cp32/18 family of supercoiled plasmids in Borrelia burgdorferi 297.* Infect Immun, 2000. 68(3): p. 1574-86.
[23] Lahdenne, P., et al., *Molecular characterization of a 6.6-kilodalton Borrelia burgdorferi outer membrane-associated lipoprotein (lp6.6) which appears to be downregulated during mammalian infection.* Infect Immun, 1997. 65(2): p. 412-21.
[24] Guo, B.P., et al., *Adherence of Borrelia burgdorferi to the proteoglycan decorin.* Infect Immun, 1995. 63(9): p. 3467-72.
[25] Parveen, N. and J.M. Leong, *Identification of a candidate glycosaminoglycan-binding adhesin of the Lyme disease spirochete Borrelia burgdorferi.* Mol Microbiol, 2000. 35(5): p. 1220-34.
[26] Fikrig, E., et al., *Arthropod- and host-specific Borrelia burgdorferi bbk32 expression and the inhibition of spirochete transmission.* J Immunol, 2000. 164(10): p. 5344-51.
[27] Barbour, A.G., *Antigenic variation of a relapsing fever Borrelia species.* Annu Rev Microbiol, 1990. 44: p. 155-71.
[28] Aron, L., et al., *Cloning and DNA sequence analysis of bmpC, a gene encoding a potential membrane lipoprotein of Borrelia burgdorferi.* FEMS Microbiol Lett, 1994. 123(1-2): p. 75-82.
[29] Lam, T.T., et al., *A chromosomal Borrelia burgdorferi gene encodes a 22-kilodalton lipoprotein, P22, that is serologically recognized in Lyme disease.* J Clin Microbiol, 1994. 32(4): p. 876-83.
[30] Akins, D.R., et al., *Molecular and evolutionary analysis of Borrelia burgdorferi 297 circular plasmid-encoded lipoproteins with OspE- and OspF-like leader peptides.* Infect Immun, 1999. 67(3): p. 1526-32.
[31] Stoenner, H.G., T. Dodd, and C. Larsen, *Antigenic variation of Borrelia hermsii.* J Exp Med, 1982. 156(5): p. 1297-311.
[32] Barbour, A.G., et al., *Pathogen escape from host immunity by a genome program for antigenic variation.* Proc Natl Acad Sci U S A, 2006. 103(48): p. 18290-5.
[33] Tabuchi, N., et al., *Immunodominant epitope in the C-terminus of a variable major protein in Borrelia duttonii, an agent of tick-borne relapsing fever.* Microbiol Immunol, 2006. 50(4): p. 293-305.
[34] Hinnebusch, B.J., et al., *Population structure of the relapsing fever spirochete Borrelia hermsii as indicated by polymorphism of two multigene families that encode immunogenic outer surface lipoproteins.* Infect Immun, 1998. 66(2): p. 432-40.
[35] Cullen, P.A., D.A. Haake, and B. Adler, *Outer membrane proteins of pathogenic spirochetes.* FEMS Microbiol Rev, 2004. 28(3): p. 291-318.
[36] Norris, S.J., *Antigenic variation with a twist--the Borrelia story.* Mol Microbiol, 2006. 60(6): p. 1319-22.

[37] Kehl, K.S., et al., *Antigenic variation among Borrelia spp. in relapsing fever.* Infect Immun, 1986. 54(3): p. 899-902.
[38] Trias, J., V. Jarlier, and R. Benz, *Porins in the cell wall of mycobacteria.* Science, 1992. 258(5087): p. 1479-81.
[39] Zeth, K. and M. Thein, *Porins in prokaryotes and eukaryotes: common themes and variations.* Biochem J, 2010. 431(1): p. 13-22.
[40] Benz, R., *Solute uptake through bacterial outer membranes.*, in *Bacterial Cell Wall*, J.M. Ghuysen and R. Hakenbeck, Editors. 1994, Elsevier Science. p. 397-423.
[41] Achouak, W., T. Heulin, and J.M. Pages, *Multiple facets of bacterial porins.* FEMS Microbiol Lett, 2001. 199(1): p. 1-7.
[42] Benz, R., *Structure and function of porins from gram-negative bacteria.* Annu Rev Microbiol, 1988. 42: p. 359-93.
[43] Benz, R., et al., *Characterization of the nucleoside-binding site inside the Tsx channel of Escherichia coli outer membrane. Reconstitution experiments with lipid bilayer membranes.* Eur J Biochem, 1988. 176(3): p. 699-705.
[44] Maier, C., et al., *Pore-forming activity of the Tsx protein from the outer membrane of Escherichia coli. Demonstration of a nucleoside-specific binding site.* J Biol Chem, 1988. 263(5): p. 2493-9.
[45] Benz, R., A. Schmid, and G.H. Vos-Scheperkeuter, *Mechanism of sugar transport through the sugar-specific LamB channel of Escherichia coli outer membrane.* J Membr Biol, 1987. 100(1): p. 21-9.
[46] Hancock, R.E. and R. Benz, *Demonstration and chemical modification of a specific phosphate binding site in the phosphate-starvation-inducible outer membrane porin protein P of Pseudomonas aeruginosa.* Biochim Biophys Acta, 1986. 860(3): p. 699-707.
[47] Kim, B.H., C. Andersen, and R. Benz, *Identification of a cell wall channel of Streptomyces griseus: the channel contains a binding site for streptomycin.* Mol Microbiol, 2001. 41(3): p. 665-73.
[48] Casjens, S., et al., *A bacterial genome in flux: the twelve linear and nine circular extrachromosomal DNAs in an infectious isolate of the Lyme disease spirochete Borrelia burgdorferi.* Mol Microbiol, 2000. 35(3): p. 490-516.
[49] Bunikis, J., L. Noppa, and S. Bergstrom, *Molecular analysis of a 66-kDa protein associated with the outer membrane of Lyme disease Borrelia.* FEMS Microbiol Lett, 1995. 131(2): p. 139-45.
[50] Skare, J.T., et al., *The Oms66 (p66) protein is a Borrelia burgdorferi porin.* Infect Immun, 1997. 65(9): p. 3654-61.
[51] Coburn, J., et al., *Characterization of a candidate Borrelia burgdorferi beta3-chain integrin ligand identified using a phage display library.* Mol Microbiol, 1999. 34(5): p. 926-40.
[52] Defoe, G. and J. Coburn, *Delineation of Borrelia burgdorferi p66 sequences required for integrin alpha(IIb)beta(3) recognition.* Infect Immun, 2001. 69(5): p. 3455-9.
[53] Coburn, J. and C. Cugini, *Targeted mutation of the outer membrane protein P66 disrupts attachment of the Lyme disease agent, Borrelia burgdorferi, to integrin alphavbeta3.* Proc Natl Acad Sci U S A, 2003. 100(12): p. 7301-6.
[54] Pinne, M., et al., *Elimination of channel-forming activity by insertional inactivation of the p66 gene in Borrelia burgdorferi.* FEMS Microbiol Lett, 2007. 266(2): p. 241-9.
[55] Barcena-Uribarri, I., et al., *P66 porins are present in both Lyme disease and relapsing fever spirochetes: a comparison of the biophysical properties of P66 porins from six Borrelia species.* Biochim Biophys Acta, 2010. 1798(6): p. 1197-203.

[56] Bunikis, J., et al., *Surface exposure and species specificity of an immunoreactive domain of a 66-kilodalton outer membrane protein (P66) of the Borrelia spp. that cause Lyme disease.* Infect Immun, 1996. 64(12): p. 5111-6.
[57] Barbour, A.G., et al., *A genome-wide proteome array reveals a limited set of immunogens in natural infections of humans and white-footed mice with Borrelia burgdorferi.* Infect Immun, 2008.
[58] Benz, R., K. Janko, and P. Lauger, *Ionic selectivity of pores formed by the matrix protein (porin) of Escherichia coli.* Biochim Biophys Acta, 1979. 551(2): p. 238-47.
[59] Kropinski, A.M., et al., *Isolation of the outer membrane and characterization of the major outer membrane protein from Spirochaeta aurantia.* J Bacteriol, 1987. 169(1): p. 172-9.
[60] Egli, C., et al., *Pore-forming properties of the major 53-kilodalton surface antigen from the outer sheath of Treponema denticola.* Infect Immun, 1993. 61(5): p. 1694-9.
[61] Benz, R., *Porin from bacterial and mitochondrial outer membranes.* CRC Crit Rev Biochem, 1985. 19(2): p. 145-90.
[62] Krasilnikov, O.V., *Sizing channels with neutral polymers*, in *Structure and Dynamics of Confined Polymers*, K. Press, Editor. 2002, Kasianowicz, J. J., Kellermayer M. S. Z., Deamer, D. W.: Dordrecht, Netherlands. p. 97-115.
[63] Krasilnikov, O.V., et al., *A novel approach to study the geometry of the water lumen of ion channels: colicin Ia channels in planar lipid bilayers.* J Membr Biol, 1998. 161(1): p. 83-92.
[64] Nablo, B.J., et al., *Sizing the Bacillus anthracis PA63 channel with nonelectrolyte poly(ethylene glycols).* Biophys J, 2008. 95(3): p. 1157-64.
[65] Krasilnikov, O.V., et al., *A simple method for the determination of the pore radius of ion channels in planar lipid bilayer membranes.* FEMS Microbiol Immunol, 1992. 5(1-3): p. 93-100.
[66] Sadziene, A., D.D. Thomas, and A.G. Barbour, *Borrelia burgdorferi mutant lacking Osp: biological and immunological characterization.* Infect Immun, 1995. 63(4): p. 1573-80.
[67] Noppa, L., et al., *P13, an integral membrane protein of Borrelia burgdorferi, is C-terminally processed and contains surface-exposed domains.* Infect Immun, 2001. 69(5): p. 3323-34.
[68] Ostberg, Y., et al., *Elimination of channel-forming activity by insertional inactivation of the p13 gene in Borrelia burgdorferi.* J Bacteriol, 2002. 184(24): p. 6811-9.
[69] Nilsson, C.L., et al., *Characterization of the P13 membrane protein of Borrelia burgdorferi by mass spectrometry.* J Am Soc Mass Spectrom, 2002. 13(4): p. 295-9.
[70] Ostberg, Y., et al., *Pleiotropic effects of inactivating a carboxyl-terminal protease, CtpA, in Borrelia burgdorferi.* J Bacteriol, 2004. 186(7): p. 2074-84.
[71] Mitchell, S.J. and M.F. Minnick, *A carboxy-terminal processing protease gene is located immediately upstream of the invasion-associated locus from Bartonella bacilliformis.* Microbiology, 1997. 143 (Pt 4): p. 1221-33.
[72] Hara, H., et al., *Cloning, mapping, and characterization of the Escherichia coli prc gene, which is involved in C-terminal processing of penicillin-binding protein 3.* J Bacteriol, 1991. 173(15): p. 4799-813.
[73] Inagaki, N., et al., *Carboxyl-terminal processing protease for the D1 precursor protein: cloning and sequencing of the spinach cDNA.* Plant Mol Biol, 1996. 30(1): p. 39-50.
[74] Trost, J.T., et al., *The D1 C-terminal processing protease of photosystem II from Scenedesmus obliquus. Protein purification and gene characterization in wild type and processing mutants.* J Biol Chem, 1997. 272(33): p. 20348-56.
[75] Pinne, M., et al., *Molecular analysis of the channel-forming protein P13 and its paralogue family 48 from different Lyme disease Borrelia species.* Microbiology, 2004. 150(Pt 3): p. 549-59.

[76] Benz, R., ed. *Porins - structure and function*. ed. G. Winkelmann. 2001, WILEY-VCH Verlag GmbH: Weinheim / Germany. 227-246.
[77] Ziegler, K., R. Benz, and G.E. Schulz, *A putative alpha-helical porin from Corynebacterium glutamicum.* J Mol Biol, 2008. 379(3): p. 482-91.
[78] Lichtinger, T., et al., *Biochemical and biophysical characterization of the cell wall porin of Corynebacterium glutamicum: the channel is formed by a low molecular mass polypeptide.* Biochemistry, 1998. 37(43): p. 15024-32.
[79] Pinne, M., et al., *The BBA01 protein, a member of paralog family 48 from Borrelia burgdorferi, is potentially interchangeable with the channel-forming protein P13.* J Bacteriol, 2006. 188(12): p. 4207-17.
[80] Skare, J.T., et al., *Virulent strain associated outer membrane proteins of Borrelia burgdorferi.* J Clin Invest, 1995. 96(5): p. 2380-92.
[81] Skare, J.T., et al., *Porin activity of the native and recombinant outer membrane protein Oms28 of Borrelia burgdorferi.* J Bacteriol, 1996. 178(16): p. 4909-18.
[82] Mulay, V., et al., *Borrelia burgdorferi BBA74, a periplasmic protein associated with the outer membrane, lacks porin-like properties.* J Bacteriol, 2007. 189(5): p. 2063-8.
[83] Pinne, M. and D.A. Haake, *A comprehensive approach to identification of surface-exposed, outer membrane-spanning proteins of Leptospira interrogans.* PLoS One, 2009. 4(6): p. e6071.
[84] Cluss, R.G., D.A. Silverman, and T.R. Stafford, *Extracellular secretion of the Borrelia burgdorferi Oms28 porin and Bgp, a glycosaminoglycan binding protein.* Infect Immun, 2004. 72(11): p. 6279-86.
[85] Mulay, V.B., et al., *Borrelia burgdorferi bba74 is expressed exclusively during tick feeding and is regulated by both arthropod- and mammalian host-specific signals.* J Bacteriol, 2009. 191(8): p. 2783-94.
[86] Thein, M., et al., *Oms38 is the first identified pore-forming protein in the outer membrane of relapsing fever spirochetes.* J Bacteriol, 2008. 190(21): p. 7035-42.
[87] Charbit, A., *Maltodextrin transport through lamb.* Front Biosci, 2003. 8: p. s265-74.
[88] Schirmer, T., *General and specific porins from bacterial outer membranes.* J Struct Biol, 1998. 121(2): p. 101-9.
[89] Barbour, A.G., *Isolation and cultivation of Lyme disease spirochetes.* Yale J Biol Med, 1984. 57(4): p. 521-5.
[90] Fraser, C.M., et al., *Genomic sequence of a Lyme disease spirochaete, Borrelia burgdorferi.* Nature, 1997. 390(6660): p. 580-6.
[91] Ferenci, T., et al., *Lambda receptor in the outer membrane of Escherichia coli as a binding protein for maltodextrins and starch polysaccharides.* J Bacteriol, 1980. 142(2): p. 521-6.
[92] Benz, R., et al., *Pore formation by LamB of Escherichia coli in lipid bilayer membranes.* J Bacteriol, 1986. 165(3): p. 978-86.
[93] Janausch, I.G., et al., *C4-dicarboxylate carriers and sensors in bacteria.* Biochim Biophys Acta, 2002. 1553(1-2): p. 39-56.
[94] Nikaido, H., *Multiple antibiotic resistance and efflux.* Curr Opin Microbiol, 1998. 1(5): p. 516-23.
[95] Koronakis, V., et al., *Crystal structure of the bacterial membrane protein TolC central to multidrug efflux and protein export.* Nature, 2000. 405(6789): p. 914-9.
[96] Andersen, C., C. Hughes, and V. Koronakis, *Chunnel vision. Export and efflux through bacterial channel-tunnels.* EMBO Rep, 2000. 1(4): p. 313-8.
[97] Bunikis, I., et al., *An RND-type efflux system in Borrelia burgdorferi is involved in virulence and resistance to antimicrobial compounds.* PLoS Pathog, 2008. 4(2): p. e1000009.